MW01155941

Praise for *The Life You Save*

"Patrick Malone has written a book that really could save a life. With his moving real life stories and his brilliant advice this book is a must-read for anyone who cares about their health and well-being."

—Sorrel King, The Josie King Foundation

"This highly practical book guides you through the essential steps for maintaining your health and avoiding medical mistakes. An invaluable resource!"

—Joan Claybrook, former President of Public Citizen

"Patrick Malone has what Pete Conrad would call 'The Right Stuff.' We owe him a debt of gratitude for focusing a beam of light on saving lives."

—Nancy Conrad, Founder and Chairman of the Conrad Foundation

"Patrick Malone has compiled a remarkably well-researched set of *you-cannot-afford-not-to* steps to take, aided by a series of life-saving checklists of questions patients need to ask, that can make the difference between getting excellent medical care or becoming a victim of impaired health, or even death, from much worse care. Doctors and other health professionals make mistakes too often to justify a false sense of security. This important book teaches patients and their families how to catch them before they cause injury or death."

—Sidney Wolfe, MD; Editor, Worstpills.org; Director, Health Research Group at Public Citizen

the life you save

Nine Steps
to Finding the Best Medical Care—
and Avoiding the Worst

Patrick Malone

Da Capo
LIFE LONG
A Member of the Perseus Books Group

FORBES LIBRARY
NORTHAMPTON, MASS.

QY.
M297L
2009

Many of the designations used by manufacturers and sellers to distinguish their products are claimed as trademarks. Where those designations appear in this book and Da Capo Press was aware of a trademark claim, the designations have been printed in initial capital letters.

Copyright © 2009 Patrick Malone

All rights reserved. No part of this publication may be reproduced, stored in a retrieval system, or transmitted, in any form or by any means, electronic, mechanical, photocopying, recording, or otherwise, without the prior written permission of the publisher. Printed in the United States of America. For information, address Da Capo Press, 11 Cambridge Center, Cambridge, MA 02142.

Designed by Trish Wilkinson
Set in 10.5-point Minion by the Perseus Books Group

Library of Congress Cataloging-in-Publication Data

Malone, Patrick.
The life you save : nine steps to finding the best medical care and avoiding the worst / Patrick Malone. — 1st ed.
p. cm.
Includes bibliographical references and index.
ISBN 978-0-7382-1304-0 (alk. paper)
1. Patient advocacy. 2. Medicine, Popular. 3. Self-care, Health. 4. Medical errors—Prevention. I. Title.
R727.45.M35 2009
362.1068—dc22 2009012690

First Da Capo Press edition 2009

Published by Da Capo Press
A Member of the Perseus Books Group
www.dacapopress.com

Da Capo Press books are available at special discounts for bulk purchases in the United States by corporations, institutions, and other organizations. For more information, please contact the Special Markets Department at the Perseus Books Group, 2300 Chestnut Street, Suite 200, Philadelphia, PA, 19103, or call (800) 810-4145, ext. 5000, or e-mail special.markets@perseusbooks.com.

10 9 8 7 6 5 4 3 2

To my wife, Vicki, who keeps me healthy

Note: The information in this book is true and complete to the best of our knowledge. This book is intended only as an informative guide for those wishing to know more about health issues. In no way is this book intended to replace, countermand, or conflict with the advice given to you by your own physician. The ultimate decision concerning care should be made between you and your doctor. We strongly recommend you follow his or her advice. Information in this book is general and is offered with no guarantees on the part of the author or Da Capo Press. The author and publisher disclaim all liability in connection with the use of this book. Some names and identifying details of people associated with events described in this book have been changed. Any similarity to actual persons is coincidental.

Contents

1

This Book Could Save Your Life

The sound patients make when they fall off the earth is so quiet that hardly anyone can hear it. For one of my clients, Richard Semsker, a forty-six-year-old attorney, the sound was a thin rustle, as his internist handed him a sheet of paper that told him his life was ruined for no good reason. He already knew that the mole on his lower back, which had recently turned a mottled blue-brown, had proven to be an aggressive cancer, a melanoma. But now the newly discovered paper told him that a dermatologist had recommended the mole be excised eight years before, long before it turned deadly. Somehow, no one had notified the patient. Richard stared at the eight-year-old letter, which his internist had resurrected from the thick jumble of papers documenting twenty years of routine internal-medicine treatment: for headaches, high cholesterol, poison ivy, and the painful boils on his back that had led to several referrals to the dermatologist. Inside, Richard was screaming. Outside, all was hushed. It would be impolite to make any noise.

So it goes with many hundreds of thousands, even millions, of Americans each year. When a person learns that a preventable medical mistake has stolen his health and that it is too late to do anything, the shock of being twice victimized—first by a curable disease and then by the caregivers who were supposed to help—causes a dizzy feeling, like everything securing him to the earth has let go. Caregivers turn from allies to adversaries.

Could this happen to you? The odds are unsettling: Medical catastrophes have been documented to so pervade the American healthcare system that a realistic risk of needless death or serious injury confronts every family in the United States at some point. But there's good news too: You can do a lot to protect yourself and to secure for you and your loved ones the best that our fragmented, expensive system has to offer.

This book gives voice to victims of bad and mediocre health care and to patients who have successfully navigated the American healthcare system. You will see how tragedies could have been averted. And you will watch as the successful patients—many of whom were victims first—enlist doctors and nurses to help them care for themselves. They clear up miscommunications before harm occurs. They persist in looking for cures when doomsayers have told them to give up. They refuse to accept "It's all in your head" and learn how to unlock the puzzles of their bodies' strange signals. They politely decline to have their bodies cut open by mediocre surgeons and negotiate access for themselves to the best surgeons and hospitals. They become literate in the statistics of their diseases and figure out how to use numbers to make wise decisions. In the process, they learn that the best way to win the longest, healthiest lives for themselves is to take charge of their own health care and not merely turn their bodies over to an impersonal and broken medical industry. "The life you save," as the novelist Flannery O'Connor once wrote, "may be your own."

To learn how to work the system, you need guidance from an expert in the system. And that's where I come in. Over the last twenty-five years, I have represented hundreds of patients and their families who lost their health to the health-care system. In each case, I've done a legal "autopsy" to figure out what went wrong with the patient's health care and why he or she was injured or killed. Before I became a lawyer, I spent a decade as a journalist covering both the best and the worst of the American medical system. In both careers, I've learned how to find the best medical care and avoid the worst. I've learned that you don't have to have a degree in medicine to understand enough to make smart medical choices. I've learned that you do need common sense, curiosity, and persistence. And you need a plan. And that's what I have put together in these pages.

American Health Care: Amazingly Good and Stunningly Bad

Americans spend more on their medical care than people anywhere in the world, by a long shot. A large chunk of that extra expense is leached out to feed the paper shufflers in the health-insurance bureaucracy, who add no real benefit. But some of the money gives us amazing technology that lets doctors peer into the deepest recesses of our bodies without cutting and perform treatments on the cellular level that would have been unthinkable only a few years ago.

Yet critics routinely describe this same health-care system as broken. Frightening statistics abound: Every year, some 100,000 people die and hundreds of thousands more are injured unnecessarily. Medical mistakes claim more lives each year than breast cancer, AIDS, and motor-vehicle crashes combined. Apollo astronaut Pete Conrad rocketed to the moon and back safely in 1969 but died of poor emergency-room care thirty years later. Medication errors alone kill more people each year than die in all the workplace accidents across the country. It's like a jumbo jet crashing every day. Arresting statistics, yes? And all of them came from a 1999 report from the Institute of Medicine, part of the National Academies of Science.[1] The authors worked hard to dress up their otherwise wonkish report with sexy, alarming numbers, and across the country the report sparked pilot projects dedicated to saving lives and reducing errors. Just the name of one project will give you an idea of the scope of the problem—the 5 Million Lives campaign of the Institute for Healthcare Improvement projected that American hospitals could save 5 million patients from harm over two years by implementing just twelve specific strategies. Five million! The same institute estimates that 40,000 incidents of medical harm happen every day in the United States.[2] These episodes can and do happen anywhere. Anyone who thinks it cannot happen to me because my doctor went to a brand-name medical school and works at a prestigious hospital is badly mistaken.

The people who cause these deaths and injuries are not evil. Nor did they necessarily graduate at the bottom of their medical-school or nursing-school classes. Many are the best and the brightest. In a way, they are victims too: of a system that has antiquated safety mechanisms and a paternalistic philosophy out of sync with twenty-first-century life, a system that propagates injury-causing errors and then does little to fix them—or even own up to them honestly.

The "Half-Nots" of American Medical Care

What may be worse than all the breathtaking errors is the inconsistent quality of the day-to-day care that Americans receive. The best estimate by quality experts is that Americans get about half the medical care recommended by consensus lists of what works and what doesn't work for the most common physical and mental diseases.[3] Half the recommended preventive care, like early screening for cancer or vaccinations. Half the care recommended for emergencies like heart attacks, strokes, and fractures. Half the care recommended for long-term issues like cancer, diabetes, high blood pressure, and depression. A grade of 50 percent is a flunking score in most schools, but in American health care, it's business as usual.

Happily for us patients, doctors and nurses across the country are doing pioneering work to figure out how to bring high-quality care to more of us (hint: it's a lot more than having a good insurance plan) and to determine how errors happen and how they can be prevented. Some hospitals are taking big steps to transform the culture of medical care to make safety and quality for patients the top priorities, to insist on accountability for results, and to be open and honest with patients when mishaps occur despite best efforts.

But unless you go to a place like the Veterans Administration for health care (yes, the VA has some of the most honest, accountable, and organized care in the country), the chance of your getting consistently excellent care with a minimum of errors is just a spin of the roulette wheel. So I will give you some tools to get out of the health-care casino and win for yourself and your family the reliably high-quality care we all deserve, care that is available virtually everywhere in the country, but that you have to work to find.

Many of us otherwise intelligent, informed adults engage in what can only be called delusional thinking when it comes to our own medical care. We read reports about how America's health indicators—infant deaths and life expectancy, to take two prominent examples—lag behind those of most other wealthy countries, and we rationalize that our own health care must be just fine and that it must be someone else's low-quality care that is bringing down the average. It's the uninsured patients, or the racial disparities in quality, we assume. The fact is that poor quality and medical mistakes are democratically distributed; we're all at risk, insured and uninsured, rich and poor, black and white. But top-quality care, indeed, some of the best in the world, is also democratically distributed in the United States and is available to everybody who has the tools to recognize the best and make sure they get it. My job in this book is to give you the tools, teach you how to use them, and motivate you for an exciting journey.

But there's one big problem we have to confront first: "We have met the enemy and he is us," as Walt Kelly's Pogo famously said. It's one thing to vow, "I will take charge of my own health care"; quite another, to put the plan into action. It can feel wrong to ask too many questions of the doctors and nurses who care for us. We have a condition we might call white-coat-intimidation-itis. The paternalistic model of health care is deeply imprinted in our psyches, for one very good reason: Sickness is scary, and everything that goes with it—needles, tubes, beeping monitors, masked humans—can be scary too. So when someone comes along in a hospital and promises to take care of us, treating us like the children we once were, it can be enormously comforting to just let go, ask no questions, and pull up the blanket snugly. Evolutionary psychologists also teach that, much as we prize our independence, deference to authority is ingrained deep in our DNA because it has proven such a successful survival strategy over the millennia. Only now are we understanding that in technologically complex, flawed systems like hospitals and clinics, deference to authority can be fatal. The point is, the time to read this book is now, before you or someone in your family faces a health crisis. And because we're all mortal, we know (but often pretend otherwise) that that crisis looms in each of our futures.

The Necessary Nine

This book is organized around the critical moments when you as a patient or as an advocate for a loved one can make a difference before it's too late. The order proceeds logically from basic building blocks to more complex issues. The safety strategy that informs the book, as you will see, starts with something the medical-care industry has begun to learn from the aviation industry: that we are all human, doctor and patient alike; that we all make mistakes; that the way we catch errors before they cause tragedy is to enlist a second and third set of eyes on whatever we're doing; and that the most effective way to collaborate on our common health mission is to boil down complex processes into simple checklists of what needs to happen and then check off the lists, item by item. Thus do we extend our lives, one checkmark at a time.

Here are the Necessary Nine steps (with their corresponding chapters):

1. ***Get your medical records, read them, and organize them (Chapter 2).*** By gathering and reading your own medical records, you will gain insight into that most fascinating of topics—yourself—and you will prevent the kind of miscommunication that led to Richard's fatal melanoma and many other preventable tragedies. It doesn't take a medical degree to help your doctors avoid tragic errors. An inquisitive mind is the main ingredient needed. This first step paves the way for every other step you need to take.

2. ***Learn how to talk to your doctor efficiently and effectively. Make a list, leave a list, and take a list (Chapters 3 and 4).*** You can plan how to talk to your doctors to give them the information they need to diagnose what's wrong with you and prescribe the best treatment. These chapters offer communication strategies to prevent misdiagnosis and arrive at the right answer—because clear communication, not fancy tests, is still the best way for you and your doctor to find out what's wrong with your body and carry through to an effective plan to deal with it. The most effective way to clearly communicate is in writing: by making a list of your concerns and symptoms; leaving the list with your doctor; and taking home another list, the doctor's action plan. When even that doesn't work and your doctor seems to be floundering, Chapter 4 offers more strategies for finding the answer.

3. ***Team up with the best primary-care doctor you can find (Chapters 5 and 6).*** What if the communication strategies you've learned from Chapters 3 and 4 don't seem to be working with your current primary-care doctor? Then it might be time to look for another one, because the ability to listen well is one of the hallmarks of a top doctor,

particularly when it comes to diagnosing what ails you. And an excellent internist or family doctor is one of your prime protectors against mediocre care and medical error. I will talk about some of the telltale tip-offs that help you scout out the best and avoid mediocre or downright dangerous doctors.

4. ***Learn the safe, sensible—and skeptical—approach to using medicines (Chapter 7).*** There are good drugs, which can save your life and ease your pains. Then there are fad drugs, useless drugs, and dangerous drugs. I'll talk about the scandal of drug-industry propaganda that too many busy doctors rely on for their pharmaceutical education. This chapter also offers practical tips for getting unbiased information about medicines and how to take them safely.

5. ***Understand why all medical tests are flawed, and seek a second or third opinion at every major crossroads of health care (Chapters 8 and 9).*** No medical test can be perfectly accurate; they all generate false alarms and, sometimes, false reassurance. In Chapter 8, I teach you how to understand the statistics behind testing error rates, so you can make intelligent choices about tests and treatments. Chapter 9 goes on to consider the related issue of second opinions. Many lives every year are saved when patients have the gumption to say, "I'd like another opinion." We're trained to think of the "second opinion" as an option only when considering elective surgery, but the concept of enlisting a second pair of expert eyes to focus on your case works for much, much more than just surgery.

6. ***Choose a surgeon by experience and team structure, and learn the checklists for safe surgery (Chapters 10 and 11).*** When you're thinking about surgery or some other major treatment, you are most vulnerable to mediocre care and error. These chapters will show you how to find the right surgeon and teach you what you must know before letting someone cut you open. I also explain the importance of check-

lists for safe surgery and how patients can improve their odds for a good outcome by checking off the key steps that doctors and nurses should do in front of the patient before they're put under anesthesia.

7. ***Have an advocate with you at every significant health-care encounter, especially in the hospital (Chapter 12).*** When you are sick, it's not only your physical defenses that are down. Your mental defenses—your ability to think things through, to exercise good judgment, to hear the advice people are giving you—suffer too. Having an ally and advocate with you at all times is the only way to go. This chapter recounts stories of injuries which an advocate can help prevent, and also shows how an advocate can spur a health-care team to give better care and get you home faster. You will also learn how to become an effective advocate for your sick family members.

8. ***Learn how to steer clear of the major hazards of hospitals and how to find hospitals that work to maximize your safety (Chapters 13 and 14).*** It's a cliché that hospitals are dangerous places, but what many people don't realize is that some are a lot more dangerous than others. Infections are such an important source of preventable injury, they deserve their own chapter (Chapter 13). Chapter 14 turns more generally to hospital quality and reviews the currently available quality-rating guides from the government, nonprofit agencies, and commercial raters. I will show why one of the most simple and down-to-earth measures—patient ratings of their satisfaction with the hospital—may be about the best.

9. ***If you develop a chronic disease, educate yourself in what you need and learn how to audit your care to make sure you get it (Chapters 15 and 16).*** The right approach to chronic disease starts with the right attitude, so I begin this final step with stories from patients who have tamed their own chronic-disease issues with determination and curiosity. Then I go on to address the uneven quality in

the delivery of care, which plagues the patients who need doctors the most. For most of the common serious medical conditions, expert specialty organizations have developed checklists that they use to audit care quality. You can use the same checklists to do your own audit, and if your care or a loved one's care comes up short, you can find a better doctor before it's too late.

Putting It All Together

Once you learn the Necessary Nine steps to finding the best health care, you'll meet some of the heroes and champions of the patient-safety movement in Chapter 17. Finally, the Epilogue gives you some steps to follow when you believe that you or a family member has suffered a needless medical injury. I will show you how to pull straight answers from health-care providers after something has gone wrong with medical treatment, so you can push the care back onto the right course. And if all else fails, I will help you figure out if you have a legal case worth pursuing and how to find the best lawyer. But my fervent hope is to generate less business for lawyers by helping readers secure the best, safest care, so you never need an attorney.

A final word: Most health-advice books are written by doctors for patients. This book is different, because I believe the experts in finding the best health care are the patients who have learned how to become their own best advocates, not so much those who dish out the care. So the advice you'll read here comes mostly from patients themselves (backed up by plenty of current scientific studies). And there's a stronger point to be made. As the Internet democratizes access to high-quality medical information, there is no reason to defer blindly to the authority of those with MDs or DOs behind their names. Doctors should be our allies, not our dictators; they should be our coaches, not our parents. Patients who take this book's lessons to heart will help make that happen for all of us, because we can help doctors see where their most effective and humane role lies.

A note about names: Many of the patients featured in this book agreed to let me use their real names. (Those who preferred otherwise had very good reasons to keep their names private.) So you will see a lot of real names in this book. On the other hand, for the most part (except when the legal cases have gone all the way to trial in a public courtroom), I do not use the real names of the doctors, nurses, and hospitals involved with injuries and deaths. This helps my publisher sleep at night, but it also underlines one of my main points. Bad things happen everywhere in our health-care system, so knowing the exact place where something awful occurred is not going to help you, the reader. What can help is to understand why and how our system doesn't work well and what you can do to patch the holes in the medical care that you and your loved ones receive.

2

Right Now: Get Your Records and Read Them

Here's the best and easiest advice for avoiding medical victimhood and attaining the best-quality health care, and it's also Step One: Get your medical records. Get them today. Read them; organize them. What you see in there may surprise or shock you, and it might just save your life.

> *Step One:*
> **Get your medical records, read them, and organize them.**

Only a few months ago, I sat across a conference-room table from Richard Semsker, a forty-five-year-old attorney, big and strong enough to have played varsity baseball in high school. His once handsome body was now bloated with the steroids he had to take for the skin cancer that had infiltrated his bloodstream and invaded his brain. Richard had recently undergone whole-head radiation, and the smooth baldness of his scalp seemed to accentuate the fine pocks of acne scars across his cheeks. I focused on his skin because it had been his undoing. Seven months earlier, his wife, Barbara, noticed that a small mole on his lower back, which had been there for years, had changed from its usual chocolate brown to a bluish mottle. Around the same time, he noticed a bump in his groin. He went to his longtime internist, who sent him one flight upstairs in the Silver Spring, Maryland, medical building, to the same dermatology office he'd visited before for skin eruptions. The date was August 3, 2006.

The dermatologist took one glance at the mole, picked up a knife, and cut it out. A few days later, the pathologist reported the worst possible news: It was malignant melanoma, the most fatal kind of skin cancer. The melanoma had already chewed deep into his skin. A couple of weeks after that, more bad news: The bump in his groin was a lymph node engorged with cancer cells. A surgeon took fifteen lymph nodes from Richard's groin, and all were positive for cancer. A scan of the abdomen found more cancer nestled near the abdominal aorta, which feeds blood to the pelvis and legs. Six months later, after a sudden spell when for a frustrating half an hour his tongue seemed to freeze and he could not speak, an MRI scan of his brain found a dozen spots of melanoma scattered like necklace beads throughout the cortex of his brain. His chance of recovery went from slim to none.

Too bad, he was told by a Johns Hopkins oncologist, the melanoma was caught so late. It's 100 percent curable when caught before it has invaded deeper than the skin.

One thought kept nagging at Richard in the months after the cancer diagnosis. He'd been to this dermatology office many times before. Two years before the grim news, in the fall of 2004, he'd had two painful cysts drained and a mole removed, all from his upper back. Between the pre-op visits and the follow-up visits after the outpatient surgeries, he'd seen various dermatologists in the practice eight times over two months. And six years before that, in 1998, he'd had another cyst on his back drained by the head of the dermatology practice, Dr. Norman Lockshin, a past president of the local society of dermatologists. Hadn't anyone seen the spot on his lower back that eventually turned deadly?

So Richard decided to ask for his records. The dermatology office sent him the 2004 records, but they had nothing for the 1998 treatment. Those records, he was told, had likely been purged after five years, the legal minimum for a Maryland doctor to retain patient records. Which meant that when he appeared in 2004, five years and ten months after the 1998 treatment, he was treated as a new patient. The dermatologist in 2004 had nothing to show him what Richard's back had looked like six years before. This dermatologist, whose name was Michael Albert, a young part-time employee of the first dermatologist, Dr. Lockshin, dutifully charted on a diagram the location of the two cysts and an "atypical nevus" (the technical term for a pigmented mole) on Richard's upper back, all of which he recommended for removal with a knife. He also drew on his diagram a line to the left lower back, where, he noted, a thirteen-millimeter "congenital nevus" and recommended regular follow-up. He wrote this in a letter to the patient's internist. No copy was sent to Richard.

By the time, two years later, Richard went back to the dermatologist after his wife noticed the color change, the lower-back mole was twenty millimeters across (a little bigger than the diameter of a dime) by twelve millimeters high. Neither husband nor wife had noticed the change in size over those two years.

But the worst news from the old records was yet to come. One evening a couple of months after the surgery to remove the cancerous lymph nodes from his groin, Richard went to his internist after office hours to see what other records about his back might exist. The internist heaved a three-inch stack of paper onto his desk and began thumbing through, page by page. "Here," he finally said, handing Richard a single sheet, "this might be what you're looking for." It was a letter from the dermatologist to the internist, addressed "Dear Larry" and dated December 1998. Dr. Lockshin reported that he had drained a painful cyst from Richard's back. At the end of the letter, he said that Richard had a "6 mm nevus" on his lower back (about the diameter of a pencil eraser), and that it should be excised.

Because the dermatologist's young employee in 2004 didn't know about the 1998 record, he assumed that the mole, which he measured at thirteen millimeters in diameter, had been stable for a long time. Any careful dermatologist who knew that a mole, even one ordinary in appearance, had doubled in size in six years would cut the mole out—without waiting to see if it turned really ugly and obviously cancerous. Richard missed this chance because the head of the dermatology practice didn't want to invest in enough file cabinets or spend fifty dollars a month for off-site storage space for old records.

Other questions crowded Richard's brain as he stared at this 1998 letter. He noticed his internist's initials scrawled across the page. Why hadn't the internist told Richard about the recommendation to take off the mole in 1998? Or at least tell him about the 2004 recommendation to have it reexamined regularly? Why hadn't the internist, who had both the 1998 and 2004 records in his file, noticed the mole's change in size?

It was outside his field. Not his job. He made the referral, and "I can only assume," he repeatedly said when I questioned him later, that the dermatologist and the patient had worked out between themselves any follow-up that was needed. That's what the internist told me when I took his deposition a few months after we filed the lawsuit.

Richard had resisted suing his internist. He called him Uncle Larry. Richard had grown up playing with Uncle Larry's son. The families lived next door. He started seeing Uncle Larry as a patient in 1986, a month before his wedding. Richard and Uncle Larry sat flank to flank at Washington Redskins games. Uncle Larry and his wife had been honored guests at Richard's twins' bat mitzvahs.

But Uncle Larry had let Richard down, and badly. He could no longer be called a friend. Worse, he had to be sued. I told Richard bluntly that no competent lawyer would file a lawsuit only naming the dermatologist as defendant. The internist's absence from the trial would create a black hole and suck the life out of Richard's case. It would be too easy for a jury to blame the absent defendant, or Richard himself, for the lack of follow-up on the dermatologist's recommendations from 1998 and 2004.

Every day across the country, fax machines and letter carriers deliver thousands of letters from specialist doctors and laboratories reporting their findings on the patients they have probed, prodded, and slid into imaging machines. Those reports are nearly always addressed only to the referring doctor. The patient who is the subject of the letter is rarely included in the correspondence. I remember how startled I was, one day five years ago, when going through the usual stack of junk mail at home, I found a letter from an orthopedist in Boston reporting his recommendations about my bad hip to my doctor in Washington. I was grateful to have been included; it's the only time that has ever happened to me. Most of the time, the reports of the specialists sail silently past us as they travel from specialist to generalist.

The idea, of course, is that the specialist will have explained her findings and recommendations in detail to us patients, and so copying us on the letter would be superfluous. Richard's dermatologist insisted, when I questioned him, that that must have happened in 1998 when he recommended removal of the then-pencil-eraser-size mole on his lower back. "I would always explain it to the patient," he said.

"One hundred percent always?" I asked.

"Well, nothing is 100 percent," he conceded.

For his part, Richard said no one ever told him to have the mole removed—not in 1998, not in 2004, not any other time—until the fateful day he went to the dermatologist again after his wife noticed the color change. Richard's medical files documented a spotless record of following up on every recommendation ever made by his doctors: every blood test, every EKG, every X-ray, every referral to a specialist. Why would he not have a mole taken off his lower back when it was the size of a pencil eraser?

These swearing contests—"We must have told you"; "No, you didn't"—could only happen in a system in which patients do not have routine access to all their health records, a system in which specialists routinely write detailed reports of their findings to the referring doctors but fail to add a critical line at the bottom of the letters: "CC: patient."

Our current system of medical record keeping combines the worst of twentieth-century technology with nineteenth-century paternalism: The technology generates lots of paper reports that take time to read, sort, file, and retrieve, all by hand; the paternalism assumes the subject of those reports, the patient, doesn't need to read them. Will the doctor's staff remember to leave the report out before sticking it in a file drawer, so the doctor can read it first? Will the doctor remember to go through the entire stack of reports on his desk? Will the doctor read all the way to the bottom of each report? Our medical system has thousands of these communication synapses—molecule-size gaps between sender and recipient. Most of the time, information is smoothly transmitted and received across these synapses, the way it's supposed to happen. But a system without backup methods of communication does not tolerate failure. So all that has to happen is for one human being to make one human mistake—to misfile, to forget to read, to neglect to mention something to the patient—and then the system comes screeching to a crash. Yet in the twenty-first century we, the patients, can fix this gap without any high-tech electronic system. We just need to read, and make sure we understand, what's being written about us.

So how do you make the system work for you?

First, you have to know your rights. The culture of medicine is so resistant to transparency (to use the latest jargon for old-fashioned candor and honesty) that you'd almost think there's a law barring patients from learning what's in their medical records. To the contrary, the law says you have every right to know. Some states go so far as to say that you, the patient, *own* your own records. And in every state, patients have a right to see every scrap of paper in a doctor's file and to have a copy made of every X-ray image (with copying charges usually assessed against the patient for the inconvenience caused to the provider).

Second, you need to appreciate why and how we can be our own worst enemies. Psychological forces make a lot of us hesitant to ask for our medical records. No one is eager for bad news, so when it comes to medical information, it's easy to assume that no news is good news. We figure that someone somewhere will let us know if we've had a worrisome test result. That's the way it's supposed to work, of course. But welcome to the real world, courtesy of medical blogger Dr. Rob Lamberts of Augusta, Georgia, who explains, "A doctor's office is always on the brink of chaos—with an incredible amount of information coming in and going out, a large number of phone calls, insurance company headaches, and personnel situations that can throw the best system flat on its face. People forget that there are hundreds of other patients with thousands of test results the office is dealing with."[1] So one rule Dr. Lamberts emphasizes: "Never assume that no news on test results is good news." Dr. Lamberts is well credentialed, with board certification in both internal medicine and pediatrics, and he runs a sophisticated, organized office with electronic medical records. So if someone like him talks about the "brink of chaos," you can imagine how much worse it is in a less well-run office.

Our internal resistance to requesting our own medical records has deeper roots than the no-news-is-good-news assumption. It's a simple enough step to ask for your own records, but it's a radical step because you are challenging authority, and that can feel wrong. Researchers have found that humans have a deep-seated attachment to the established and the familiar, even when it can be shown that established ways threaten our very survival.[2] That explains why societal systems like communism and apartheid can hold the allegiance of their subjects long after any rational outsider can see the system is broken, and it also explains why we persist in trusting an antiquated medical communication system long after we know that something better is needed.

All of the above is to say that I don't minimize how hard it can be to take this first step of the nine steps I advocate for taking charge of your own health care. If you put it off, if you wait until a health crisis confronts you, it will be far more difficult to take this first step, because our natural tendency to cling to the familiar becomes stronger the more threatened we feel. So it will never be easier than it is right now. And I can predict one more thing: If you try this first step, you will find that obtaining, reading, and organizing your own medical records will lead you naturally to the other steps necessary to take charge of your own health care. It will become second nature to ask questions, to evaluate, and to make informed decisions that maximize your chances of a long, healthy life.

How to Obtain Your Records

So here is some specific advice about how to get the job done and what to do with your records to make them useful for yourself and your doctors. Obtaining your own medical records is only slightly more difficult than falling out of bed. The easiest thing to do is to ask for the record from each provider the next time you're in that office. You may have to sign a form that talks about your privacy rights under the Health Insurance Portability and Accountability Act (HIPAA). You may also have to pay a per-page fee for the copies. But the provider must give you a copy, usually within thirty days under federal HIPAA regulations.

Here's a form letter you can use for requesting your records. This was put together by the Georgetown University Center on Medical Record Rights and Privacy. It's a little legalistic, and you don't necessarily have to get this elaborate in your request, but it does do the job.

Sample Letter to Request Health Records

[Your name]
[Your address]
[Date]

[Name of care provider or facility]
[Address]

RE: [Your medical identification number or other identifier used]

Dear ———,

The purpose of this letter is to request copies of my medical records as allowed by the Health Insurance Portability and Accountability Act (HIPAA) and Department of Health and Human Services regulations.

I was treated in your office [at your facility] between [fill in dates]. I request copies of the following [or all] health records related to my treatment.

[Identify records requested (e.g., medical-history form you filled out; physician and nurses' notes; test results; consultations with specialists; referrals).]

I understand that you may charge a "reasonable" fee for copying the records but will not charge for time spent locating the records. Please mail the requested records to me at the above address.

I look forward to receiving the above records within thirty days, as specified under HIPAA. If my request cannot be honored within thirty days, please inform me of this by letter and provide the date by which I might expect to receive my records.

Sincerely,
[Your signature]
[Your name printed]

Under HIPAA you can be charged a "reasonable" fee for copying records. You may also be charged for postage if you ask that records be mailed to you. HIPAA allows thirty days for a provider to respond to your request for records, with one thirty-day extension for good reason. HIPAA also allows you to request a summary of your medical records. If you prefer a summary, you should agree to a fee beforehand. Your state laws may include a smaller fee for copies of records or a shorter time for the provider to respond to your request. The Georgetown University Center on Medical Record Rights and Privacy includes state-specific guides for thirty-two states.[3] Before composing your request for medical records, visit their Web site for information about your state.

Organizing Your Records into a Personal Health Record

Getting your medical records is only the first step to making them into something useful. You don't want to show up at your next doctor's appointment with a wad of paper sticking out every which way. That's guaranteed to win you the ten-foot-pole treatment.

An organizational scheme will also help you educate yourself as you're sorting through the papers. Here's what will be most useful to you and your doctors:

1. A chronological set of all your blood and urine tests. This can show important trends over time.
2. A chronological set of all imaging studies—plain X-rays, MRI, CT scans, and the newer PET scans—on various parts of your body. It's ideal to have a disk with the images themselves, and most radiologists now can give you a disk at minimal cost. But at a bare minimum, you should collect and save copies of all the official reports on any imaging studies.
3. Records of all surgical procedures you've had. The best thing to keep is a copy of the official operative report, plus any pathology report on tissue removed during the operation. The anesthesiologist's notes are also potentially helpful, because they can show if you've had any problems with anesthesia.
4. A list of all your current medications and dosage schedule. You can get this from your pharmacy (but the list may not show the dosage instructions). Never use more than one pharmacy at a time for different medications. Pharmacies have software programs that check for medication conflicts, and you want to give these programs a chance to work.

For more guidance, see the Web site of the American Health Information Management Association.[4]

There are ways to use software or the Internet to compile a personal health record. Microsoft and Google both have products in this space. As you might expect, those two are the big players in organizing your medical records via the Internet. But there are many other services, either free or for a small fee. Go to the Nursing Online Education Database for an excellent article by Alisa Miller, which describes the pluses and minuses of all the Web-based services to help you acquire and organize your medical records.[5]

Two more tools will help you decipher your records:

- A Web site, Lab Tests Online (http://www.labtestsonline.org/), lets you look up any of the thousands of clinical lab tests and find out what they mean and how to interpret your results.
- A dictionary of medical abbreviations translates cryptic acronyms into English; some of these you can get from an Internet search, but a good comprehensive dictionary is Neil M. Davis's *Medical Abbreviations: 30,000 Conveniences at the Expense of Communication and Safety,* 14th ed. (Warminster, PA: Davis Medical Abbreviations, 2008).

One Small Step, One Giant Leap: A Patient's Success Story with His Records

Here is one patient's story of how he became an informed and involved patient, starting with his own medical records. Tony Benedi became an expert patient, not by choice, but because he had to if he wanted to stay alive. In February 1993, Benedi, a short, stocky Cuban American who had just finished a stint as a White House aide to the senior George Bush, came down with what he thought was the flu. He took Tylenol several times a day for the aches. Within a few days, he had sunk into a coma with what doctors diagnosed as a near-fatal reaction to the Tylenol. He had to undergo an emergency liver transplant. His kidneys were damaged too, and a decade later, a nurse, who had befriended Tony while he recovered from the liver transplant, donated one of her kidneys so he could come off of dialysis. Living with someone else's liver and yet another someone's kidney and taking a fistful of pills every day to prevent rejection of the transplants is enough to turn anyone into a near doctor of their own body. What's more, Tony and his wife Maria's two college-age sons both suffered testicular cancer in the space of less than a year. So Tony Benedi has had a lot of dealings with doctors and hospitals.

Tony's journey toward becoming an informed and active patient started with the simple step of insisting on seeing his own laboratory-test results as they came off the printer. Tony has to have his liver and kidney blood markers monitored every few weeks to look for early signs of damage to or rejection of the transplanted organs. At first, the laboratory refused to send the test results directly to Tony. The lab would fax them to the doctor's office, and the report would sit in the doctor's in-box for a few days. Meantime, Tony would be stewing and wondering what the results were. Finally, Tony got the doctor to intervene with the lab, and now Tony gets lab results within an hour after the blood is drawn.

Getting the records leads naturally to Step Two (discussed in depth in our next chapter), talking to the doctor. When Tony spots something out of whack in his lab report, he calls the doctor, and they decide together what to do. You have to build a relationship with your doctor before you reach this point of smooth teamwork, Tony says. In his case, it helped that on a prior occasion he had spotted something the doctor had completely missed—his liver enzymes, a marker of liver-cell death, had shot up. When Tony pointed it out and questioned what it meant, more tests were done, and they found that the lab results were an early sign that the duct carrying bile from the liver was clogged up. The doctors went in with a balloon and cleared the blockage before any damage was done. Tony's eagle eye on the lab sheet helped make the treatment happen in time. It's not that the doctor is a bad person for overlooking the out-of-whack lab number; it's just a lot easier to find and act on an abnormality when the doctor is backstopped by a second set of eyes with only one patient's lab numbers to worry about.

The watchword for Tony's involvement in his own health care has been "polite but persistent." Tony is an inquisitive person. He asks questions. He keeps asking questions until he understands. Because he's a regular guy, not a medical genius, sometimes he has to ask a lot of questions. He says of physicians, "They're not gods, they're human beings. The more the patients know and ask the doctors, the more the doctors are receptive in accepting patients' involvement in their own care."

Tony offers another tip for patients first venturing into self-advocacy: *Get involved with a patient group.* Tony found that meeting with other patients with similar problems helped him and others to break through the intimidation of asking questions of someone wearing a white coat. Says Tony, "It's helpful to have another patient tell you that, yes, you can ask that question. And then you find out, there are alternatives to everything. You get three doctors together and they all disagree. So my attitude now is, once they stop saying that they're 'practicing medicine,' then maybe I'll take their word for it. But as long as they're 'practicing,' I'll ask questions."

Raising Your Doctor's Game

Readers who follow the model of Tony Benedi, and other patients whom you will meet later in this book, will win a bonus: better all-around care. Here's how Dr. Andy Thomson, a Charlottesville, Virginia, psychiatrist, put it when we discussed the nine steps of this book: "When doctors know they are dealing with an informed patient, they 'raise their game.' They do better. It's just like when you're playing pickup basketball and somebody really good wanders onto the court. When the doctor knows you're looking over his shoulder, the reality is he will pay more attention to your case and be more careful. That's fundamental human nature."

Of course, it can also be human nature to feel defensive when someone invades your turf. "If you ask persistent, polite questions and the doctor reacts adversely, that says something negative about the doctor, not about the patient," says Dr. Thomson. That could be a signal that you need to find another doctor. I will talk more about this in Chapter 5.

A Glimpse into the Future

Some health-care systems in the United States have eliminated the cumbersome part of this book's Step One. They have put their patients' records onto secure Web sites that patients can access with a few clicks. If you are a patient of the Veterans Administration or another leader in the electronic medical-record revolution, such as the Marshfield Clinic in Wisconsin or Brigham & Women's Hospital in Boston, you are ready for the interesting part of Step One: reading and understanding your medical records and then asking questions.

Even in those systems, the medical-record integration only goes as far as the boundaries of the institution. If you get care from anywhere else, special steps have to be taken to stitch those records into your other records. That, too, is starting to happen in some places. The benefits of a fully integrated medical-care record, to which patients have easy access, are hard to overstate. Eventually, these systems will integrate your current internist's records with all specialists and labs, now and forever: an entire life of seeing doctors combined into a single electronic record. Every prescription you've taken, all the important numbers—every blood-pressure and every cholesterol reading, every single lab test you've ever had—and with pictures, to boot: every tooth X-ray, every biopsy slide, every cardiogram, all the shadows, the swirls of microscopic cells, the squiggles of your heart rhythm across the page, everything. And you, the patient, will be able to see everything on an Internet site where you can control who else gets to see your data. In one fell swoop, this will fix much of the brokenness of our current health-care system: the fragmented care, the left hand not knowing what the right hand has prescribed, the tragic communication errors like the one that killed Richard Semsker. Even better, integrated electronic records allow doctors at places like the Marshfield Clinic in Wisconsin to pool information about thousands of patients to do research on what works and what doesn't work.

The system that armed-services veterans enjoy is one of the furthest along. Veterans can see all their records at http://www.myhealth.va.gov. But the system is still clunky and hard for doctors to use. The software was cobbled together in the early 1980s—pre-Windows, pre-Mac—by some doctors working in the basement of the Veterans Administration Medical Center in Washington, D.C. They in turn relied on various pieces—a pharmacy program here, a radiology package there—that had been created by amateur programmers at VA clinics around the country. It's not a pretty system, but it works. The program is called VistA. It is at the heart of a quality revolution that has wowed health-care insiders. Veterans' hospitals and clinics don't just deliver more integrated care than just about anywhere, but they can prove with hard numbers that veterans get better results, fewer complications, and fewer medical errors. It's not just easier in the veterans' system for patients to monitor their own care and doctors to coordinate with each other. What's more, administrators can collect data that is anonymous for individual patients but "provider specific," so they can pinpoint what surgeons have the lowest complication rates, and what primary-care doctors are doing the best job for their chronic disease patients, and a bunch of other data that has made veterans' care such top quality.[6]

Unless you're a veteran or a patient at one of the few other institutions that integrate all their care records, you have to deal with our current fragmented system, although perhaps not for too many more years. President Obama's economic stimulus program, announced in January 2009, included a proposed $20 billion to computerize all Americans' medical records, but it faced a big fight between the health-information industry, which promotes ease of access to medical records, and consumer groups, which want strict protections so consumers can control who gets to see their most private and sensitive information.

Until these debates are resolved and we have a national electronic record system in place, you have to construct your own integrated care record. A daunting task, but it's not hard to do when you take it one step at a time. It's crucial that you start asking for a copy of everything, every time you go to the doctor or lab. Now, when you ask for a copy of your radiology report or your lab test, be prepared for the quizzical look, or even a dose of red tape. But do not give up. And take comfort that you are a pioneer making it easy and routine for all patients who follow you.

Lifesavers:

Your First Steps for the First Step of Getting and Reading Your Own Records

Gathering and reading your own medical records is an essential first step to becoming an informed, proactive patient. You should especially get a copy of every lab report, X-ray study, and specialist's report. The easiest way to take the first step of this first step of our Necessary Nine steps is to start asking for these routinely, up front, when you're about to have the test done. Take with you a standard form, already filled out and signed, and leave it at the front desk. When you see how easy it is to get your results, and how it's not hard to understand them (most of the time), you can then go back and start to pick up all your old records so you can put them together into a good chronology. Your doctors will appreciate it, and you'll learn a lot about your own health.

3

Talking to Your Doctor: Put It in Writing

Have you ever felt that your doctor just wasn't listening to you? Or that he'd made up his mind about what was wrong with you when you'd barely opened your mouth? This chapter develops a strategy for getting your doctor to really listen and pay attention to you. I call it Step Two of the Necessary Nine: *Learn how to talk to your doctor efficiently and effectively. Make a list before you arrive, leave a list with the doctor, and take a list home.*

> *Step Two:*
> **Learn how to talk to your doctor efficiently and effectively. Make a list, leave a list, and take a list.**

An amazingly high percentage of medical conditions can be diagnosed by astute doctors from the patient's story alone. High-tech imaging scans and exotic blood tests can confirm the diagnosis, but the key clues are the observations about our bodies that you and I carry around with us and relate to our doctors, before they lay one hand on us. After all, the human brain is the processing end of a highly sophisticated and sensitive system that monitors the body's internal workings, and much of the time, it far outperforms medical gadgetry in providing early signals that something is going haywire. That's why it's important for each of us to give an accurate history and for the doctor to listen and absorb the story. But many things stand in the way of a good history soaking into our doctors' heads, and therein lurks potential tragedy. That is why improved communications are important not just for respect between doctor and patient, but to reduce your chance of being misdiagnosed and mistreated. In this chapter you will also learn much of what you need to know to decide if you should stick with the doctor you already have; we will talk more about choosing a doctor in Chapter 4.

Meagan's Story

Meagan Moran (not her real name) was in many ways a model patient. A bright, cheerful, sandy-haired woman in her mid-forties, Meagan had achieved a master's degree in health administration and had run two busy doctor's offices, even helping her orthopedic-surgeon boss write speeches and raise money for his nonprofit foundation. She left the workforce to have children but still managed her daily life with precision and attention to detail. She made lists and schedules for her and for her husband and two children. She entered them in a neat, small script in pencil in a Day Timer notebook. When things were done, she put a check mark on the list.

And when she felt sick on a Wednesday just before Easter, Meagan made another list, dutifully recording all her symptoms with a mechanical pencil in her neat script on a sheet of lined notepaper. She first recorded her recent history: The prior weekend, she'd had what she assumed was a vaginal yeast infection and had treated it with an over-the-counter drug but was still very irritated in that area. Monday and Tuesday, she had some pain below her rib cage and an episode of dark urine. But what prompted her to sit down and record all this on a

Wednesday just after lunchtime was what she felt at 11:30 AM that day: "sudden onrush of radiating pain lower back, both sides," with "chills, weak neck down." And just below a reminder to pick up her kids from school, she wrote, "Had vag strep once before. Am I contagious?"

Meagan went to her internist early in the afternoon of that same Wednesday. We know, from what she wrote and what she told her husband later that day, that she was puzzled and worried about the sudden stab of pain in her lower back. She had a strong, healthy back, and hadn't bent or twisted or lifted anything that could explain this pain. Plus, she had what she thought was the yeast infection in her vagina, or was it vaginal strep?

The internist did a short examination and assured her that most likely she was experiencing the first pangs of the flu, even though it was April, well past flu season. He did a pelvic exam and concluded that the irregular red rash on her vulva came from a yeast infection. He wrote prescriptions for a flu medication and an antifungal drug for the vaginal infection. He advised Meagan to go home, stay in bed, get plenty of fluids, and take the medications for what he assumed were two unrelated problems.

Only she didn't have two unrelated conditions, but just one: streptococcal bacteria in her vagina that was starting to invade the deep tissues and produce back pain. The Monday after her Wednesday appointment, after dutifully following the doctor's advice for five days, and after speaking to his medical partner on the Sunday night, she returned to his office, so weak that her husband had to enlist a security guard with a wheelchair to take her from the car to the doctor's suite in the medical building. The internist couldn't get a blood pressure. He called 911. She was taken to a nearby hospital. All her organs were overwhelmed by the poisons produced by the strep bug, and even though she received intensive treatment, she died the next day. The final diagnosis: streptococcal toxic-shock syndrome. She was forty-six years old. And so Meagan joined the swollen ranks of patients victimized by an overly optimistic medical diagnosis made without carefully listening to the patient.

When Cheerful Assumptions Can Kill

Research says that as many as 15 percent of all medical diagnoses are wrong.[1] Any misdiagnosis causes wrong treatment. But tragedy lurks in one distressingly common type of misdiagnosis: the assumption that the patient has a benign, self-limited condition, when in reality the clock is ticking on a treatable serious disease that could kill if left untreated.

Ordinary penicillin could have tamed the group A *Streptococcus* bug that killed Meagan. It is one of only two or three bacterial strains that never developed antibiotic resistance.

There was plenty that the internist left out in his hurry to make a diagnosis. He took no culture of her vaginal discharge, did not check her urine, which she had told him was a dark color, and did not draw any blood to see if her white count was elevated (a sign of bacterial infection, not the viral flu that he assumed). But most of all, he didn't listen to the whole story she told him. Instead, he picked out the parts that fit his preconceived idea of flu.

No one was in the exam room but the internist and Meagan. So how can we know he ignored pieces of her story? Because after she died, her mother found the sheet of paper from her Filofax day planner on which, in her neat, small script, Meagan had listed her symptoms before going to see the doctor, including her prescient final thought: "Had vag strep once before. Am I contagious?" She had drawn an arrow in the margin pointing to that last question. Her husband had seen her writing this list on her way to the doctor's office.

None of these items in her notes made it into the doctor's record of the visit, which he tapped out on a laptop computer. Why not? Either he hadn't heard what she said, or he hadn't asked her the thorough questions, body system by body system, that would have teased out her full story.

In the lawsuit that I brought against the internist on behalf of Meagan's two children and widower, the internist tried to blame her for his not hearing the full story on that spring afternoon in his office. If he was right, then this patient, a Phi Beta Kappa college graduate with a master's degree in health administration, had written out her history and symptoms just before the examination, but then had deliberately withheld the information from him during the exam. That seems unlikely. And while we'll never know exactly what words were exchanged during the appointment, I think we can easily reconstruct how the miscommunication occurred. Meagan's symptoms and worries that she wrote to herself did not penetrate the doctor's consciousness, because of a common logical error that afflicts all of us when we sort out reality: Out of the jumble of perceptions we take in, we seize on what fits the pattern our mind wants to find, and we discard the rest. Usually we go with what fits our experience and preconceptions. This is called confirmation bias.

Confirmation bias is not always a bad thing. Experience shapes wisdom, at least some of the time. But truly wise doctors know that a patient's illness may not fit into their preconceptions, so they are open to new information from the patient. And their training warns them of the peril of discarding pieces of the patient's story. Yet because the vast majority of the patients a primary-care doctor sees in any week will have something benign and self-limited, doctors have a natural tendency to assume that the next patient on the schedule also has something benign. And that bias is a threat to any patient like Meagan, who has a truly serious condition.

Doctors are taught to ask an open-ended question when they first encounter a patient, something like, "What brings you in today?" Just as important as the question is the listening that is supposed to come next as the patient relates their problem, in their own words, without interruption. But researchers who observe doctor-patient encounters report that the ideal is seldom met. One study of the University of Chicago's hospital emergency room found that while most doctors started with an open-ended question, four out of five patients were interrupted before finishing their answer. The average time until interruption: twelve seconds.[2]

Communication is especially important for primary-care doctors, the first to encounter a patient's new problem. A now-classic study from Oregon published in the *Journal of the American Medical Association* in 1997 found that, comparing never-sued primary-care doctors with those who had at least two claims against them, the never-sued doctors spent more time with patients, used more humor, and used specific tactics to facilitate communication, such as asking patients' opinions, checking understanding, and encouraging patients to talk.[3] That doesn't make them perfect, just more likely to hear the patient's full story and thus steer toward a more accurate diagnosis.

When I took the deposition of the doctor who misdiagnosed Meagan's vaginal infection, he was stiff, cold, and superior. He didn't need to test what her vaginal infection was, he said, because he could tell by a glance. A test would have wasted time and money. Meagan's handwritten note came up only indirectly in the interrogation. I asked him if it wasn't true that she would read her symptoms from her notes in the doctor's office, something her husband had seen on other occasions. He said, "I don't specifically recall that." He also said he couldn't say if she was a "good historian," because he had no way of corroborating if she had forgotten, overstated, or understated any of her pertinent history. He admitted, though, that she had "excellent comprehension" and was "a very nice person whom I enjoyed having as a patient."

So how did this very nice person end up with a body bloated with fluids that her lungs couldn't clear and her kidneys couldn't process, which finally caused her heart to shut down? Her internist was not a "bad doctor." He certainly didn't fit the clichéd image of the malpracticing doctor addled by drug or alcohol addiction or old age. He just didn't listen well and thought he could guess his way toward the correct diagnosis rather than use any of the diagnostic tests at his disposal.

Leaving the List: A Simple Step That Could Help Your Doctor and Save Your Life

Meagan had already done more than most patients to take charge of her own care, by writing down her symptoms and organizing her thoughts before going to the doctor's office on that fateful Wednesday. But she could have done one more simple thing: She could have handed her notes to the doctor and asked him to read them and put them in his office chart. This would have confronted him directly with all the symptoms that didn't fit into his glib flu diagnosis, and could well have moved him toward taking her condition more seriously.

My friend Lew Stoneburner, a successful malpractice lawyer in Richmond, Virginia, has seen too many miscommunications turn into tragedy. So any time he is feeling bad enough to see a doctor on a nonroutine basis, Lew types out a list of his symptoms and takes it to the doctor's office. He hands it to the nurse and asks the nurse to put it in his chart. He then makes sure to talk over the list with the doctor.

Beth McGlynn, a leader of health-care-quality research at the RAND think tank in California, goes to her internist with an index card. "I write down a list of things I want to talk to her about, because I don't trust my own memory," Dr. McGlynn told me. "She's been seeing me for twenty years, so she knows we're not going anywhere until we check off every item on the card."

Smart health-care consumers all over the country are following a system like this. Here's what graphics guru Edward Tufte, a retired Yale professor who specializes in clear communications, usually with pictures, says on his Web site,

> In advance of the meeting, the patient prepares a typed-out list of all the issues to be covered at appointment with the doctor. This list should include causal speculations by the patient: "This pain on my right side might be a gall bladder issue. A grandparent and my father had gall bladder problems around my age." The patient should make several copies of this list-agenda paper and bring them to the appointment.
>
> At the beginning of the meeting, the patient hands a doctor a copy of the list. The doctor, who did not get to be a doctor by being a slow reader, can read about 3 times faster than the patient can talk. After handing the agenda-list over, the patient should

> look down at her/his own copy, hinting that it is time to start reading. Or perhaps saying, "Here it all is, read this."
>
> . . . The list gets everything the patient initially has to say out on the table, without interruption. As the appointment continues, the list helps set an agenda and a schedule for the allocation of time during the meeting. It also helps to make sure that the patient does not abandon lower-level issues that should be discussed—because there the issues are, already written out. Each item on the list is, in effect, checked off as the appointment moves along. Perhaps the patient should even ostentatiously check off the first point on the list after it is discussed to indicate that this list is what we're going to march through. The idea is that the doctor is not only going to be looking at the computer and at the patient, but also at the list. Because the patient keeps looking at the list.
>
> The patient should bring several copies of the list to the appointment, since the patient may see several medical staff members during the appointment. Each medical person gets the agenda-list. For example, my doctor often has a medical student in training who handles the initial discussion and who then goes off to describe the situation to the doctor, who shows up later. Both the student and the doctor get copies of the agenda list.
>
> The list-agenda enhances the efficiency, accuracy, and resolution of the information presentation made by the patient. It also helps reduce socially or situationally-determined answers to the doctor's questions; instead some of the patient information has already been prepared in advance, free of social pressure.
>
> This list goes into the patient file and also assists the doctor in preparing notes for the patient record. Maybe someday the patient provides the list via email in advance of the appointment; even so, the patient should still bring paper copies to the appointment itself.
>
> —Edward Tufte, April 12, 2005

More recently, *New York Times* columnist Jane Brody recommended arriving for a doctor's visit with a written list of concerns and symptoms.[4] This is one way to cope with the fact that the average time allowed for patient encounters in many medical offices is down to seven minutes.

The extra step that I advocate, leaving the list with the doctor, is intended to defeat confirmation bias and thereby increase the accuracy of diagnosis and treatment.

Better to Win Respect Than Love

List making, list presenting, list focusing: It doesn't sound like a way to ingratiate yourself with your doctor or her office staff. Yes, this technique will risk getting yourself branded as a "pain in the rear end" patient. But you're not looking for their love; you're looking for competent health care. And being a focused, organized patient will win your doctor's respect, and gratitude too, because you will make their time with you more productive and efficient. Plus, remember that it's all in the presentation. If you thoughtfully write your list and present it in a low-key but persistent way, with plenty of smiles and other warm signals, you can bet that thoughtful, mature doctors will appreciate the way you have made their job easier. Nobody wants to misdiagnose a treatable condition and cause a tragedy like Meagan's.

Here's another reason why you want to be very sure that everything important you tell your doctor gets into the doctor's written record. When key facts don't make it into the medical record, the usual assumption afterward is that the patient must not have communicated the information. Victims of medical error discover too late an unwritten rule of malpractice litigation: The doctor's record becomes the official history of what happened because it was written at the time. Juries tend to distrust a patient's after-the-fact protestations about what was said, especially if the doctor's notes look thorough and careful. This frustrates injured patients and their families. "You mean if he doesn't convict himself by his own records, he gets off?" many clients have asked me incredulously. "Not exactly," I say. "But you need some corroboration for your version of what happened. His version is the record he made when he saw you. That can be hard to attack." I also explain to clients that independent evidence can come from other sources: other doctors' records, lab studies, the observations of honest third parties like nurses, or in Meagan's case, her own handwritten notes—all can provide important clues that a doctor's records are incomplete or downright wrong. But if the patient wants to be a good witness for his own case, there is no better way to do it than to write the symptoms and present them to the doctor before miscommunications and misunderstandings cause malpractice. And if that nips the misunderstanding and makes for better care, then so much the better, because no patient wants to trade good health for the consolation prize of a malpractice lawsuit.

Making a Good List for Talking to Your Doctor

The list you take to your doctor's office should try to answer these questions:

1. What is my top concern? Why did I make this appointment?
2. What else about my health concerns me?
3. What are my symptoms?
4. For each symptom: What seems to bring it on? When did it start? What made it go away? How often does it happen? Does it happen at a certain time of day or night, or in connection with a certain activity? What else have I noticed about the symptom?
5. What changes in habits or routines have I had lately?

Be concise. You're making a list, not writing a short story. Using too many words defeats the whole purpose of accurate yet quick, complete yet efficient communication.

You should also have a standing list that you give your doctor, which includes the following:

1. All medications, over-the-counter drugs, and supplements you're taking, including the dosage and dosing schedule.
2. A complete list of all doctors and other health-care providers whom you are seeing, including their phone numbers and e-mail addresses.

If You Can't Make a List . . .

What if there's no time to make a list? You're on the way to the emergency room. The last thing you have time to think about is list making. There's a second-best remedy: Take someone with you to any nonroutine interview with a doctor, especially when it's a new problem. The person who's not having the crisis is in the best position to make sure the doctor gets a clear and complete story of what happened. Another reason why this is important is because a psychological defense mechanism sometimes kicks in that makes it hard for us to give a fully accurate story to the doctor. It's called denial. Males are especially susceptible. The chest pain? The numbness down one arm? I cannot be having a heart attack. Not me. It must be indigestion from that burrito I just ate.

Having an advocate with you is so important that it's Step Seven in our list of the Necessary Nine steps for better health care. The discussion here will be expanded in Chapter 12, which focuses on the importance of having an advocate with you when you are hospitalized overnight.

Your Advocate Is Your "Bodyguard"

The person who accompanies you to the ER or doctor's office has multiple functions:

- They help you keep your story straightforward and complete.
- They listen on your behalf to what the doctor says.
- They write things down.

- They ask questions.
- They make sure they understand, so that you understand.
- They keep you grounded in reality.

Remember, you may think you're Superman or Superwoman, but that's right now, when you're reading this book and life is swimming along just wonderfully. When you suddenly find your body turning against you, producing scary and strange feelings, you are not likely to react with the level of rationality that you need to make the best decisions.

Another Critical Moment: Leaving the Doctor's Office

I've talked about the importance of walking into the doctor's office with a written list of questions and problems. There is one more list of equally critical importance: the list you take with you when you leave the doctor's office. That list is the action plan. You should try to get as much of this as you can in writing. It prevents misunderstandings. So think of it this way: in with a list, out with a list.

At a minimum, the take-home plan of action needs to include these answers:

1. What tests are to be done? Why for each one? How will the results change the treatment? (If a test is being done just for the doctor's curiosity, it might be better not done.)
2. What medications are to be started? Why? For how long?
3. What should you notice about the results of the medication, and when should you see it? Are there common side effects you need to watch out for? (Every medicine has side effects.) Are there any tests you need to monitor the drug's progress or to look for early signs of bad side effects?
4. What medications are to be stopped? Why?

5. What kinds of problems should you be on the lookout for before the next appointment? Whom should you call if you have a problem?
6. When is the next appointment?

These moments at the end of the appointment are crucial. You have probably waited a long time to see the doctor. You're eager to go home. The doctor wants to move on to the next patient. Don't let any of that stand in the way of your understanding the answers to all these questions. Without a clear understanding of the action plan, you have set yourself up for failure.

Trying to Reach Your Doctor: "I'm Sorry to Bother You, But . . . "

One more issue we should discuss in this chapter is our natural hesitation to call our doctors outside business hours (which is, of course, when all the really bad stuff happens). How many times have you prefaced your remarks when calling a doctor with these words: "I'm sorry to bother you, but . . . "?

Dr. Faith Fitzgerald, a Sacramento, California, physician and teacher of internal medicine, wrote an essay in *Annals of Internal Medicine* in 2008 about how hard it was for her to convey a message to another doctor about a patient they shared. The whole maze of telephone voicemail was set up to make it difficult to reach any human being and impossible to actually get the doctor on the phone. Everyone assumed the doctor didn't want to be bothered. She was struck, when thinking about it, how invariably when a patient called her, they always started with, "I hate to bother you, but . . . ."

Dr. Fitzgerald wrote, "I tell my patients, residents and students that they should call me if they need me. They are not an interruption to my work; they are my work. In this sense, I can't be 'bothered' by them. But a system and a culture designed to protect doctors from their patients assume I am bothered, and so gives that same impression to those trying to reach me. This really bothers me."[5]

Janice47, a hospice nurse, wrote this advice to the *New York Times* blog Well, in response to a story about Dr. Fitzgerald's essay:

> My recommendation to people? Call, call back and keep calling (but not for trivial things like giving antibiotics to parakeets). Remember who is paying the bills for the services they render to you. You are. You would not allow such behavior from other service industries; your waiter or your car specialist or your hairdresser, would you? You can always change MDs. You can send written complaints. People are afraid to push since they feel they won't get good care or that the MD will not take care of them any longer. That is simply not true in most cases. As long as you are calling about things regarding your health (or others) that cannot wait, you should be answered. And if you have chest pain and trouble breathing, for goodness' sake, call 911. Many people call MDs for things that the MD can do nothing about in the office anyway. Some die waiting.
>
> Like I always tell my patients, be the squeaky wheel.
>
> —Posted by Janice47[6]

Practical Advice for When the Question Cannot Wait

If you need to reach your doctor and are having trouble getting through, the following suggestions will help:

1. Ask for the doctor's nurse or physician's assistant or nurse practitioner. Many times they can answer your question or get the doctor to call you back faster than if you just leave a message for the doctor to call you back.
2. Fax your question to the doctor.

3. E-mail the doctor. (E-mail addresses can sometimes be dug out from the doctor at a face-to-face meeting or from a resume posted on a Web site, or an article the doctor has written.)
4. Be persistent but polite. If you don't hear back within twenty-four hours, consider switching to another doctor.
5. Don't abuse your doctor's good will. Contacts outside regular hours should be limited to problems that seem urgent.

One Alternative to Calling Your Doctor at Night

One final piece of Meagan Moran's story needs to be told at this point. She took the flu medication her internist gave her for five days, and then on a Sunday evening when she felt no better (and had had a fever spike to 104 earlier that day), she called his answering service and received a call back from his partner. He told her to take over-the-counter medications to reduce the fever and her back pain, and call the office in the morning. This was tragically mistaken advice. By the next day she was in shock from the strep infection, and it was too late. He should have told her to go to the emergency room. But it raises a question that all of us have faced: Should we go to the emergency room? Or just try to handle it on the telephone?

The problem with telephone advice is the doctor cannot see you and examine you. In Meagan's case, what made it worse is she was talking to a virtual stranger, her internist's partner, who didn't know her and wasn't familiar with her last visit to the office. That is a setup for misunderstandings. Dr. Joy Lewis, a careful, compassionate internist in Jackson Hole, Wyoming, agrees with Dr. Faith Fitzgerald's lament that patients should not worry about "bothering" their doctor on the telephone at such times. But she adds this advice for such circumstances: "A general rule, if you are sick enough to call a doctor with your illness complaints in the middle of the night, early morning, or on a holiday (times you may not wish to 'bother' the doctor), then go to the ER. You are therefore sick enough to be seen and evaluated by someone. I can tell you as a doctor receiving these calls, I, too, do not feel 'bothered,' but I do think, *They are calling me at a time when they 'don't want to bother me,' so something is wrong—more likely than not.* The ER can either figure it out or reassure them and me."

We all know that emergency rooms are not fun places to be, especially in the middle of the night. But if it's worth making a phone call, it may be worth the trip.

Lifesavers:

Key Tips for Taking Step Two for Effective Communications

To communicate effectively and efficiently with our doctors, the best strategy is to take a list with us to the doctor's office and leave it with the doctor to become part of the chart. See pages 38–39 for the five items (plus two more) that should be on that list. Then we should be sure to take home with us another list—the action plan. See pages 40–41 for the six questions that list should answer. Having an advocate-ally with us for the visit is another key element for clear communication and understanding. If we need to reach the doctor outside regular hours, there are several tactics that work to get through (see pages 42–43), but remember that if it's urgent enough to reach the doctor immediately, it could well be important enough to make a trip to the emergency room.

In the next chapter, we will take our communication strategy one step further for those critical times when our doctor doesn't have an answer for what ails us.

4

When the Diagnosis Is in Doubt

So you have followed my advice in the last chapter, and you have had a good, full discussion with your doctor. All your cards have been placed face up on the table with your written list of problems and symptoms that you have handed over. Now it's her turn. What does she think is wrong with you, and what does she propose to do about it? You're listening intently. And instead of certainty and confidence, the doctor places a wild card on the table. It could be a lot of things. She doesn't really know. But she thinks you'll be fine. It's probably . . . nothing.

Right at this moment, you can help your doctor and possibly save your own life with one simple question:

"Doctor, what else could it be?"

This question is not for every visit. But it's a great, important, life-saving question when

- the doctor obviously hasn't fit all the pieces of the puzzle together (particularly as in Meagan's case, when the patient has developed simultaneous symptoms that might fit into one diagnostic box and the doctor wants to parcel them out into two or more unrelated boxes);

- the doctor is unsure about what's wrong but tries to reassure you that it probably is nothing to worry about; or
- the doctor has seen you multiple times, and your body isn't responding to his or her treatment plan.

This simple question is seldom asked, and therefore even less often answered. But it could be the most important question you'll ever ask a doctor. It could be your ticket to helping prod the doctor out of complacence and to take your condition seriously.

Why do we seldom ask, "What else could it be?" It can seem a rude and impertinent question to put to someone in a white coat. But there's a deeper problem that makes many of us hesitate to ask. Especially when the diagnosis offered is benign, it's a lot easier to embrace a vague pronouncement like "probably nothing" than to entertain the idea that something bad may be lurking undiscovered within ourselves, something that might rear up and kill us. Who but a hypochondriac would challenge the diagnosis of "probably nothing"? Objectively, of course, we know we will die someday, and we know that our own denial of that can land us in a lot of trouble. Every year, thousands of heart-attack and stroke victims delay going to the hospital until hours after their first symptoms, even though they know that delay could kill them. No, they insist, it's just a passing pain. That's why a vigilant spouse can be a real lifesaver.

Yet when patients have conquered their own natural denial and delivered themselves to a medical facility, doctors are sometimes all too willing to exert, often unconsciously, their own denial that this patient could be having a life-threatening problem. It's the job of the health-care professional to take the patient seriously. A doctor who looks first for a benign source for the patient's symptoms rather than for those things that can kill the patient does no service to the patient.

We don't go to doctors to feed our natural instinct for denial. We go to doctors to make sure that something really bad isn't happening to us, and if it is, to find the right treatment to make it better. Why do people go to "emergency" rooms? To see if there's an emergency!

The question, What else could it be? is intended to prod the physician into a thinking exercise she learns in medical school: the differential diagnosis. Here's how it works. The physician takes the patient's significant findings and makes a list of all the diseases that could fit. The list is supposed to be prioritized to put dangerous treatable conditions first. Often, though, the doctor makes a probabilistic diagnosis as a shortcut. Just like Meagan Moran's internist did with her. Something similar cost my client Sharon Burke part of her brain.

Sharon Burke's Story

Sharon Burke was a successful retail menswear store manager in the Washington, D.C., suburbs of Prince George's County, Maryland. She was forty years old, single, and popular with her friends for her quick wit and positive outlook. In December 1999, Sharon Burke underwent an MRI scan of the brain because she had started experiencing strange symptoms: numbness and tingling of her arms and legs, mostly on one side. The scan was reported by radiologists at Groover, Christie & Merritt, a large Washington, D.C.–based group radiology practice, as showing signs of multiple sclerosis, a degenerative disease where nerves lose their insulation sheathing.

The symptoms went away, and Sharon Burke's neurologist did nothing until she came back to him in July 2000, seven months later, complaining of similar symptoms. This time the symptoms were more dramatic: She had had episodes where one of her legs suddenly gave way and she fell. She also had short spells of numbness in one or the other leg. Another MRI scan was ordered. This time the report was more equivocal. The radiologist said the scan looked like Sharon Burke might have multiple sclerosis, or an inflammation of blood vessels in her brain, or as a third and last possibility, a stroke from a blood clot.

The radiologist misread Sharon Burke's brain scan. The July scan actually showed a blockage of one of the major blood vessels feeding the brain—the right internal carotid artery—and clear evidence of stroke damage in the parts of the brain fed by that artery. Sharon Burke went on to suffer a major stroke several months later, a stroke that could have been prevented if her scan in July 2000 had been read correctly and she had been put on aspirin or other medications to block the development of the clots that injured her brain.

The incorrect brain scan report by Dr. William Higgins of Groover Christie misled both Dr. Stuart Goodman, Sharon Burke's neurologist at the time of the scan, and another neurologist, Dr. David Moore, to whom Sharon's mother took her in September 2000, frustrated by Dr. Goodman's failure to figure out what was wrong with her. Both neurologists ordered a series of tests to chase down the possibility of multiple sclerosis and other diseases, which Sharon Burke didn't have. Ironically, the second neurologist looked at Sharon Burke's brain scans himself just a few days before she suffered a major stroke, realized that they showed an artery blockage, and scheduled her for more tests on her blood vessels that would have finally produced the correct diagnosis—but the orders came too late.

On the morning of October 23, 2000, Sharon's mother, Wilhelminia Torian, came to Sharon's condo, in a suburb just east of Washington, D.C., to pick her up for the test on her blood vessels. She found Sharon sitting in an easy chair in her bedroom, staring into space, unable to speak or move. An ambulance took Sharon to a hospital, where imaging tests found the blood clots in her neck arteries and the arteries in the brain. But it was too late to prevent major brain damage. Sharon Burke lost the ability to think clearly, to walk normally, and to speak more than a few halting words. Her career in sales was ruined. She has to depend on her elderly mother to run those parts of her life that most of us never think about: shopping, paying bills, housecleaning.

Four years after that, our lawsuit against Sharon's doctors reached the courtroom. I still remember the hollow rattle when I picked up a bottle of aspirin and showed the jury that a simple medication could have prevented her tragedy. But what could Sharon and her mother have done differently so that we didn't have to go to court?

Several things they clearly did right. For instance, when the symptoms came back after a seven-month reprieve, Wilhelminia started attending all her daughter's medical visits. That's a smart strategy (and it's Step Seven on our list of the Necessary Nine steps—more in Chapter 12). For someone who's sick and bewildered by their own body's new and foreign signals, it's too much to expect that one person to be able to competently report everything wrong and to ask all the right questions of the doctor. Sharon and her mother also did the right thing when they fired the first neurologist once it was clear that he was bewildered by Sharon's condition.

One thing that Sharon and her mother could have done that might have halted the cascade of errors that led to an unnecessary stroke would have been to ask a simple question, What else could it be? That would have led to a discussion of the possibility of stroke. After all, stroke was on the radar screen after the second MRI in July, when stroke was listed as the third of three possible causes of her condition on the erroneous MRI report. Those mini episodes where Sharon's leg gave way or suddenly turned numb, and then cleared up in an hour, all those could easily be explained as mini strokes, or what doctors call TIAs (for transient ischemic attacks; ischemia is what happens when any part of the body loses its supply of oxygen-rich blood). And the doctors could have explained to Sharon that the weeks just after a TIA are the highest-risk time for a major stroke. And they could have explained that stroke is much more readily nipped in the bud than multiple sclerosis, which has no cure, or the blood vessel–inflammation disease that they also speculated she might have. Of the three possibilities listed on the radiologist's report, stroke was the only urgent one to check out: urgent because it could cause sudden, devastating injury, not just slow deterioration like the other possibilities, and urgent because something could be done about it if the cause of the stroke could be pinpointed.

Sharon's "mistakes" were entirely innocent: First she fell into the hands of a mediocre neurologist who had no coherent plan for figuring out what was causing her episodes of sudden numbness and weakness in her arms and legs. Then she was sent to a mediocre radiologist who missed the key evidence of a blood clot blocking one of her major brain arteries. Then she found a new doctor who did have a plan but with the wrong priorities. Sharon never knew how urgent her situation was. Only careful and persistent prodding by Sharon or her mother could have pushed the neurologist into acting faster and to refocus first on the life-threatening, urgent possibilities of what was wrong with her.

Tricia Torrey: One Patient's Success Story

In 2004, Trisha Torrey was a fifty-two-year-old former elementary-school teacher turned self-employed Internet marketing consultant, living in Syracuse, New York. Trisha raised two daughters as a single mother after a divorce in the 1980s. In late June 2004, she found a golf-ball-size lump below the surface of her skin on her upper abdomen. It didn't hurt—it was just there. She saw her family doctor the next day; he sent her to a general surgeon who removed it the same afternoon in an office procedure. He told her he would call when he had the results from the lab about what the growth was. Two weeks later, the surgeon called. Trisha remembers his exact words: "You have a very rare cancer—a lymphoma—called subcutaneous panniculitis-like T-cell lymphoma." Then he told her that the lab results had taken two weeks because the outcome was so rare that another lab had been called for a second opinion. "Two labs have independently confirmed these results," she was told. "We'll make an oncology appointment for you as soon as possible." That took another two weeks. Meantime, she hit the Internet.

The name of the condition itself was a clue to the diagnostic problem. The name said it was a lymphoma—a cancer of the lymph glands—that was "like" panniculitis, which is an inflammation of the subcutaneous fat. In short, a cancer that looked like something completely benign.

Subcutaneous panniculitis-like T-cell lymphoma—SCPTL for short—is an aggressive killer, Trisha learned. Most patients live no more than a couple of years—with or without treatment. Trisha relates what happened next:

"When I finally saw the oncologist, he was very discouraging. Dr. S., I'll call him, sent me for blood work and a CT scan, both of which came back negative for any abnormalities. No sign of lymphoma. And I had no symptoms to speak of—at least in my estimation. Okay, so I had night sweats and hot flashes, but hey! I was a fifty-two-year-old woman! Don't we all? But Dr. S. insisted that those were symptoms of lymphoma and I needed to think about chemotherapy—and soon. Without chemo, he told me, I would be dead before Christmas. I asked about the possibility that the lab results were wrong. No—not a chance. Two labs had independently confirmed the results."

Still, she put off a decision. Now July had rolled into August. Trisha learned that her first oncologist was sick, and his partner, Dr. H., had taken over. She spoke to him on the telephone and told him she was thinking about getting an opinion from another oncologist. Dr. H. said flatly, "What you have is so rare, no one will know any more about it than I do." That made Trisha mad, and she resolved to dig deeper. A friend gave her the name of another oncologist, Dr. Jeffrey Kirchner, who happened to be treating someone else with this rare lymphoma. Dr. Kirchner offered to see Trisha. Trisha then got copies of all her records, including the reports from the two pathology labs that had supposedly independently verified the diagnosis.

It turned out that neither pathologist had reached any definitive diagnosis. The first one had written in his report that Trisha's fatty tissue contained streaks of lymph cells "of uncertain significance, suspicious for a T-cell lymphoproliferative process." That pathologist sent the slides to a more specialized pathologist, whose report stated that her cells were "most consistent with" and "highly suggestive of" SPTCL, but that a further study would be done of "clonality," to see if the cells were reproducing themselves as cancer cells would.

Worse, her oncologist had no copy of the "clonality" report that supposedly would confirm that this was a terrible cancer and not an inflammation of fatty tissue. When Trisha prodded the doctor's office, they finally acquired the clonality report from the laboratory. The report was negative. Her cells were not cloning themselves.

Meantime, she saw Dr. Kirchner, who told her that even if she had SPCTL, it would be better treated with radiation than chemo. He recommended that they send all her biopsy slides to an expert at the National Institutes of Health, Dr. Elaine Jaffe, a pathologist with special expertise in T-cell lymphomas.

Three weeks later, Dr. Jaffe confirmed that Trisha had no cancer, only plain, vanilla panniculitis. She has had no problems since then. But that's not the end of the story. Trisha was angry at her first oncologists for pressing her so hard to undergo chemo when they hadn't even seen the results of the clonality study. She found online case reports of other patients who had been diagnosed with and had undergone chemo treatment for SPTCL and who had died as a result, only to have an autopsy show they had never had the disease.

Trisha wrote letters to all the doctors involved, praising those who had straightened out the misdiagnosis, blasting those who had caused it. She wanted them to understand what it meant for a patient to receive news that she had a fatal disease and needed immediate, aggressive treatment, only to find out it wasn't so at all. She received a defensive letter from Dr. H., the oncologist who had insisted she needed no second opinion. She had a more positive interaction with the chief pathologist at the second laboratory, who explained in an e-mail exchange how the misdiagnosis could have occurred. Then, a few years later, Trisha found herself at a medical conference where this pathologist was on a panel. She introduced herself afterwards. Trisha says, "We shook hands, we even hugged—and he proceeded to tell me about all the changes they have made in his lab, based on the procedural holes uncovered during my diagnosis. I was floored. He thanked me for my post-misdiagnosis follow-up that exposed the problems. He invited me to visit the lab. And then he apologized." She felt a flood of relief and wept in the car all the way home.

The experience of uncovering her own misdiagnosis changed Trisha Torrey's life, and probably saved other lives as well. She sold her marketing company and became a full-time patient advocate. As she says, "I'm a spiritual person. I believe everything happens for a reason. And so I am here today advocating for others. I'm doing my best to turn those misdiagnosis lemons into empowerment lemonade. Granted, my anger still creeps into my work on occasion. But I know I'm helping patients empower themselves, so that 'edge' may be somewhat helpful."

Now, after successfully negotiating the medical system, Trisha is remarried to a wonderful man with whom she travels and plays golf. She gardens and works in stained glass when it's too cold for golf. She has a good life—and a better one, since she took charge of her own care. The only reminder of her misdiagnosis is an ugly four-inch scar on her abdomen. The best thing, she says, is this: "I now know why I was put on this earth. A pastor friend of mine calls it Trisha's calling."

Trisha Torrey built a Web site full of tools for patient empowerment at http://www.diagknowsis.org. She writes newspaper columns, hosts a radio show, teaches workshops, responds as an expert on another Web site, and is writing a book. You can read more about her at her blog, Every Patient's Advocate, at http://trishatorrey.com.

Lifesavers:

Critical Questions to Ask Your Doctor (Step Two, Continued)

When the doctor isn't quite sure what you have, or when he seems a little too sure for the circumstances, or when you've tried the recommended treatment and it's not helping, these are the critical questions you need to ask:

1. "What else could it be?"
2. "Is there any chance that I have a condition that can be treated now but if not caught soon, could be a disaster? If so, how do we get to the bottom of that?"
3. "Are there any of my symptoms or test results that just don't fit your diagnosis? If so, what else could be going on?"
4. "You say I've got two separate, unrelated things wrong with me. Is it possible there's just one thing wrong that explains all my symptoms?" Or,
5. "You say you've found one thing wrong with me. But that doesn't explain all my symptoms. So is it possible I've got more than one thing going on?"

Also, remember the checklist of questions, on pages 40–41 at the end of Chapter 3, about the action-plan list you should take home when you leave the doctor's office. Those same questions apply when the diagnosis is in doubt, and even more so.

5

Your Best Ally: A Top Primary-Care Doctor

Many people think they automatically get better medical care by skipping the general-practice doctor and going straight to a specialist. This is a common misconception. These same people would never dream of doing a major renovation on their house without a general contractor to coordinate all the subcontractors. The problem is, before you are really sure what's wrong with you, and especially if you have more than one thing wrong with you, when you skip past the primary-care doctor you are setting yourself up for misdiagnosis, for batteries of needless and expensive tests, and for injury from those tests.

> *Step Three:*
> **Team up with the best primary-care doctor you can find.**

This happened to a friend recently. When she developed abdominal pain that persisted, she went to an emergency room and from there to a gynecologist; both she and the emergency doctor assumed that one of her female organs was causing the pain. She underwent multiple surgeries where the gynecologist used a telescope stuck through a slit in her belly button to try to find what was wrong with her uterus or fallopian tubes. It turned out her appendix was inflamed and needed to be removed. An internal-medicine doctor would have saved her the trouble of the gynecologic surgeries by sending her to a general surgeon.

Primary-care doctors—now mostly internists and family-practice doctors—serve a critical function that too often gets overlooked and even maligned in a society that values the exotic and the specialized. They are the frontline diagnosticians; they examine the entire patient head to toe; they can diagnose most of what ails us and can steer us to an appropriate specialist for what they cannot diagnose. Then they serve another critical function when we go from specialist to specialist: They are the coordinators of the care, and the repositories of the data generated by the various specialists and consultants. That's why Step Three of our Necessary Nine says, "*Team up with the best primary-care doctor you can find.*" And I placed this step *after* the one about learning how to talk to your doctor because it may turn out you already have a top primary-care doctor. One of the best ways to determine the quality of your current doctor is to try the communication strategies suggested in the last two chapters with your current primary doctor. If he or she responds with enthusiasm to your written lists of problems and symptoms, and if he or she seems to listen well, you may already have the primary doctor you need. But if you have any doubt or hesitation about your current primary doctor, read on.

Sotiri's Story: Too Many Specialists, Too Little Primary Care

Sotiri Ponirakis was an athletic junior-college student with dark good looks and a penchant for practical jokes. He worked summers in his dad's construction business in northern Virginia. When he was a senior in high school, Sotiri had noticed blood in his urine once, then seemed healthy for a couple of years, then developed protracted bouts of vomiting that left him so dehydrated that he'd faint. Soon he was having episodes of stabbing pain somewhere between his heart and stomach. Each time, at his internist's referral, Sotiri went to specialists. A gastroenterologist put a scope down his stomach and took a piece of it for a biopsy. An emergency room ran blood tests. A cardiologist had him undergo a stress test on a treadmill, then put a catheter into his heart and took pictures of the coronary arteries. He even had some knee pain, for which the internist sent him to an orthopedic surgeon. All of them reported back to the internist: nothing wrong with the heart, nothing wrong with the stomach, nothing wrong with the knee. Only some disquieting lab results, indicating widespread inflammation in his body and some abnormal kidney function. These results fell outside their specialties, so the specialist doctors assumed the internist must have noticed and heeded them. They were wrong. The internist never did his job of taking charge of the patient's overall care to figure out why this twenty-year-old man was having so many strange ailments.

Then one day Sotiri had a renewed attack of pain, this time focused on his flanks. New tests showed that his kidneys had been destroyed. He had to start dialysis immediately to clean the waste from his blood. The kidney specialist, a bright, cheerful man named David Mahoney in Fairfax, Virginia, looked back at Sotiri's old records from all the testing he underwent. There he found repeated signs that the kidneys were going south. Creatinine, a protein that the kidneys normally clear with great efficiency from the blood, was elevated to twice normal on repeated tests. The internist had never noticed, because he had not ordered the tests. The specialists who first saw the test results forwarded them on to the internist thinking he would take charge, since the kidney was not in their domain. Since no one was in charge, Sotiri Ponirakis lost his kidneys to a treatable disease—an autoimmune disorder called lupus nephritis, in which the body attacks itself, thinking its own cells are foreign invaders.

A few years later, I lost too. I presented Sotiri's case to a jury in Fairfax, Virginia, and because they concluded that the internist owed Sotiri no more than the referral slips sending him to the specialists, the jury voted against Sotiri and for the internist. The jury was wrong. I blame myself because I assumed they knew more than they did. I thought everyone knew that a patient's internist always stays in charge of his or her patient's case and is always supposed to coordinate care and coordinate specialists. The jury instead bought a glib story from the defense lawyer that the internist does enough if he reacts to each symptom by sending the patient to a specialist in the general area where the symptom came from. Pain near heart, send to cardiologist. Pain in knee, see orthopedist. Pain in upper abdomen, stomach specialist.

Real internists know better. They are not just ticket writers who send patients to this and that specialist. They are in charge of the entire insides of a patient (and the skin too), and they stay in charge even when they send the patient for specialist referrals. You must know and appreciate this, or something like what happened to Sotiri could happen to you.

The Primary Doctor: Medical Detective, Coordinator, and Lifesaver

When patients like Sotiri Ponirakis don't have a primary doctor who takes on the job of staying in charge, coordinating the care, and using their diagnostic skills to figure out what is wrong, patients fall through the cracks of the medical system. The same thing happened to Richard Semsker, the skin-cancer patient you met in Chapter 2.

Richard had seen the same internist for twenty years. By the time I met this internist, he was pushing eighty years old: a kindly looking, jowly old man. His records made it clear that at one time he had taken seriously the job of being care coordinator, because he had a front sheet on Richard's record, where he listed all the specialists he had sent Richard to over the years and a few words about their diagnosis and treatment. This sheet is called a problem list. Every internist is supposed to have one for each patient. It's a shortcut for keeping track of a patient's problems, and it saves a busy internist from having to leaf through many pages of old records to compare new reports with old reports to make sure nothing significant has changed.

In Richard's case, something significant did change, but the internist didn't notice, because he hadn't kept his problem list up-to-date. In 1998, Richard had seen a dermatologist, who recommended that a six-millimeter mole on the lower back be excised; then in 2004, another dermatologist in the same practice spotted a thirteen-millimeter mole in the same place and assumed it was a birthmark that didn't need to be removed. The second dermatologist didn't know about the old record, so didn't appreciate that the mole had doubled in size in six years. The internist had saved both records in Richard's file but never compared them.

At a deposition four weeks before Richard's death, I confronted his internist with the ethics manual from the American College of Physicians. The doctor confirmed that he was a member. But he didn't recall ever reading the ethics manual. Here's what it said:

"A complex clinical situation may call for multiple consultations. One physician must remain in charge of overall care, communicating with the patient and coordinating care based on information derived from the consultations. Unless authority has been formally transferred elsewhere, the ultimate responsibility for the patient's care lies with the referring physician."[1]

Eventually the internist agreed with the ethics statement, but he also said, "I discharged my duty" when he made the referrals to the dermatologists and never kept up his problem list.

Richard Semsker sat beside me silently as the internist gave this testimony. He later said how alone and abandoned he felt when he learned that his internist wasn't really the coordinator that Richard had always assumed he was. Richard Semsker ultimately paid with his life for the lack of coordination between his internist and the dermatologist.

To keep this from happening to you, you need a clear line of communication and understanding with your internist or family doctor, whoever is going to be in overall charge of your care. It's a partnership.

You're the homeowner. The general contractor is your main doctor. There may be times when you feel like you should be your own general contractor. If you've had a disease long enough, you may feel that you know more about it than your doctor. If so, it's time to move on to a doctor who knows more than you. You're not just paying them to be your prescription-writing machine.

Lest you think there is anything radical in my account of the way it's supposed to work, consider what a group of top leaders in medical-care quality agreed was the top priority for the system at large: "Patients must be at the center of the care system and have the right to coordinated quality care."[2]

In 2007, the leading primary-care doctors' organizations—representing pediatricians, family practitioners, internists, and osteopaths—put out a document called the "Patient-Centered Medical Home," which calls for fundamentally changing the fragmented health care most of us receive. The idea of the doctors' groups is to organize care around a "medical home" in which each patient has an ongoing relationship with a personal physician, who is in charge of a team that provides comprehensive, coordinated care with quality and safety hallmarks like electronic medical records and software that tells the doctor automatically what the latest research shows about the patient's condition. And the "medical home" also will have expanded hours and easy ways for patients to communicate with doctors, such as via e-mail.[3]

A Checklist for Finding the Best Primary-Care Doctor

How do you find and latch on to a primary-care doctor who takes seriously his or her job as your partner in the health-seeking adventure? And how do you make sure that this same doctor is focused on safety and quality? I've put together a checklist of questions to ask and clues to look for. I say "clues" because every primary-care doctor is going to pay lip service to what you want to hear; the proof is in the way the practice actually works, which you will only discover from other patients or hard experience.

You can bypass a lot of these questions, at least for the time being, if someone close to you is medically sophisticated, knows your local area, and is tuned into your proactive patient philosophy. There is no finer recommendation than finding out where doctors or nurses send their family members for primary care. (As we will discuss in Chapter 10, the same applies for surgery, but only if your endorser has inside knowledge of what operating-room professionals observe.)

First, is the doctor board certified in either internal medicine or family practice? (Or pediatrics, if you are shopping for a child.) This certification means the doctor has sat for a rigorous full-day written test (plus an oral exam for surgeons). And the boards that administer these tests are now requiring doctors to be retested every dozen years or so to keep their certifications. (Older doctors don't have to undergo recertification.) You will see the certificate on the office wall, or you can just call the office and ask, or you can check online. Warning: Besides the twenty-four specialties (and more than a hundred subspecialties) approved and certified by the American Board of Medical Specialties,[4] there are other specialty "boards" that may have far less rigorous requirements. It's a free country; any group of doctors can get together, come up with a name, call themselves the American Board of XYZ, and declare that anyone who pays annual dues and shows up for meetings in nice resorts is certified by their board. So don't just ask if your doctor is board certified, ask, "Board certified in what?" There's nothing necessarily wrong with a doctor having one of these less traditional board certifications, but if that's *all* she has, a large red flag should go up in your mind. The ABMS Web site can tell you if a doctor is certified by any of its twenty-four boards.[5] Note: Osteopathic physicians (DO) have their own certifying boards,[6] but they are as rigorously trained as MDs.

Second, is the doctor subcertified in a specialty board for your medical issue? If you are in absolutely perfect health, this question doesn't apply, and in fact, you may be better off with a generalist who doesn't have any specialty focus, because you are seeing him for his diagnostic, big-picture skills. But if you have any kind of long-term issue that falls in the domain of one of the subboards under internal medicine, you would be well advised to find a doctor in that specialty. There are eighteen subspeciality certificates issued by the American Board of Internal Medicine, from familiar ones like cardiology, rheumatology (arthritis), geriatrics, and endocrinology (diabetes), to less well-known ones, like sleep medicine. (You can see the full list at the board's Web site.[7]) Now, many board-certified internists who do not have one of these specialty boards will still regularly see patients in these domains, so this is not a hard-and-fast rule. But when your issue is management of a long-term problem, you're usually better off with a specialist in that problem.

Third, find out how accessible the doctor is outside of scheduled appointments. What is the system? Does she respond to e-mail? Are you expected to talk to a nurse first? (Not necessarily a bad thing, I should add; you just need to know the system.) After hours, would the callback come from the doctor personally or from some backup doctor who may know nothing about you?

Fourth, and this is especially important for a primary-care doctor, how well does he listen to you? Are you discouraged after trying the communications pointers from Chapters 3 and 4? If so, it's time to move on. But note also, this is item four on our checklist, not item one. It's a big mistake to put communications skills ahead of basic training. The medical knowledge has to come first.

Fifth, does the doctor show some compassion and empathy for you, without being condescending? Cold care is bad care. Even if the care is technically proficient, you need to see someone with whom you have some emotional connection, because trust and confidence help the therapeutic relationship as much as any technical know-how. For one thing, a good relationship encourages you to follow the doctor's advice. If you leave the doctor's office feeling stupid or that you've wasted her time, that doctor is not for you. At the same time, you want to be treated like a grown-up.

Sixth, does the doctor address what really scares you, even if you haven't fully put it into words? People often go to the doctor out of fear. You might be having recurring headaches. You mention the headaches, but you don't mention that you're really worried about brain cancer or a blood vessel in your head bursting open. Any doctor who doesn't have the sense to realize that you're not there just to be told to pick up some over-the-counter headache pills is not for you.

Seventh, does the doctor tell you more about the doctor's own problems than you need to know? If you start telling your doctor your problems and you wind up hearing a long discourse on how something similar happened to him, you might wonder if you should charge for the visit, not the other way around. Some doctors try to be more "human" with their patients and "relate" to them by telling the patient lots of stuff about the doctor that the patient doesn't want to know or need to know. Professional boundaries need to be respected. If this is a frequent problem with your doctor, go elsewhere, because it's a sign that the doctor isn't putting you first.

Bottom line, you have to find a doctor you can trust and relate to. That is not to undercut this book's advice. One excellent internist, Dr. Rob Lamberts of Augusta, Georgia, puts it into perspective: "Please note that trusting a doctor *does not mean you should not ask questions.* In fact, I think a physician who does not want to be questioned is one you should *not* trust. Questioning is often the only way to build trust. Unanswered questions tend to undermine trust."[8]

A Few Final Checklist Items for Your Primary-Care Doctor

I would also look for these things in a primary-care doctor:

- The doctor has at least a few years experience after passing the board-certification exam.

- The doctor has admitting privileges at a good hospital. (See http://www.qualitycheck.org for hospital ratings and Chapter 14 for an explanation of the different hospital-rating systems.)
- The doctor works with at least one other well-trained and well-qualified doctor in the same specialty who provides backup when he or she is not available.
- The doctor has a neat and comfortable office, with reasonable waiting times.
- The doctor has a stable practice with no recent, unexplained moves.

Lifesavers:

Your Guide for Step Three: Finding a Top Primary-Care Doctor

A top primary-care doctor is your best guide and partner on your health-seeking journey through life. This doctor should be your frontline detective in finding out what's wrong with you, developing sensible preventive-care strategies, and monitoring the work of the specialists to whom she sends you. Finding a good primary doctor starts with matching your care needs with the doctor's training credentials, and then focuses on his or her listening and explaining skills. See the other key questions to ask a prospective primary-care doctor on pages 61–63.

6

Steering Clear of Dangerous Doctors

Some very smart patients think that to find a good doctor, it's enough to check out the negatives: Look up lawsuits and disciplinary actions by the state licensing board, and if the doctor comes up "clean," that must mean he or she is worthy of your trust. And if that same doctor shows up in a local magazine's annual list of "best doctors," that seals the deal. I wish it were that easy. Here's the real truth:

- Lawsuits are only a crude barometer of quality. One or two lawsuits against a doctor don't necessarily amount to a black eye, especially in a specialty that attracts lawsuits because injuries tend to be so bad (such as obstetrics and neurosurgery, where brain and spinal-cord injuries sometimes happen, even with acceptable care).
- Just because you don't find any lawsuits in an Internet search doesn't mean that the doctor hasn't quietly settled a string of horror shows out of court. So a "clean" rating on lawsuits really means "unknown."

- State licensing boards, which are supposed to take away the licenses of the very worst doctors and enforce quality standards for the rest of the profession, are notorious for being slow, inefficient, and protective of the profession they are supposed to regulate.
- Those "best doctor" lists you see in your local glossy magazine are popularity surveys that have about as much thought and reliability put into them as your office's "March madness" basketball pool.

Thirty years ago, I worked on a team of reporters and editors at the *Miami Herald* on an exposé series about "dangerous doctors" in Florida. These doctors had behaved so outrageously, even criminally in some cases, that they deserved never to practice medicine. Yet practice they did for many years, thanks to an overworked state licensing board that saw its job, once it got around to a specific case, more as a counseling agency, focusing on forgiveness of the wayward practitioners and reconciliation with the medical mainstream. The series caused a furor, won our team a bunch of journalism awards, and helped usher in more of a consumer-protection philosophy at the state licensing board. But I can't count the number of times I've felt Yogi Berra's "déjà vu all over again" in the three decades since, as I've seen headlines about lax medical discipline all over the country. One of the most recent jaw-dropping cases involved a surgeon named John Anderson King, DO, who, despite a string of problems in other states, moved to West Virginia in 2002, started doing spinal-implant surgeries, racked up in six months of practice more than a hundred lawsuits against him and the hospital that hired him, and then . . . moved on.[1] He was later spotted working at a family-practice clinic in Alabama (with a new, legally changed name), then in Orlando, Florida. If you try to look him up on the West Virginia board's Web site, you will find nothing.

When you do find a practitioner's name on an official list of license discipline, chances are that the discipline will be for drug or alcohol abuse or sexual misconduct. Those are the easy cases for the state licensing board. It doesn't take a *Law and Order* prosecutor to pull the medical license of a doctor who's been convicted of drunk driving, or stealing narcotics from an operating-room supply cabinet, or fondling a patient's genitals. But when competence is at issue, only the most flagrant cases get a licensing board's attention. And what might seem flagrant to you or me might not look so bad to a licensing board, especially when the board likes to cut a break for the doctor. Knowing how hard it is to get the attention of the state regulators, I have filed complaints in only a handful of cases with the Maryland Board of Medicine for what I thought was outrageously poor medicine. In the most recent, the board finally told me that the surgeon whose overdose put a client of mine named Helen F. (last name withheld at family's request) into a lifelong vegetative state was issued a "private reprimand." I couldn't even find out what the board said in its letter, because, they informed me, private reprimands are private; the public has no right to learn a thing about them. If you look up this surgeon on the state's official Web site, it says "none" under disciplinary actions, "none" under malpractice judgments, and "none" under malpractice settlements. Each of those I know to be false.

This same surgeon is listed among the "top doctors" in the Washington, D.C., metropolitan area by our local glossy magazine, the *Washingtonian.* So are several of the other doctors I've sued over the years on behalf of patients. The *Washingtonian* says it compiles its listings from a random survey of thousands of local doctors. Don't get me wrong. Reputation is a wonderful thing. It's just not enough to assure yourself that this is someone you want to trust your life to.

Lanh Martin's Story

Lanh Martin (her name has been changed), a lovely Vietnamese American who had two children in grade school, went to a "top doctor" listed in the local magazines, after her own mother had suddenly developed advanced liver disease and then died within a month of the diagnosis. Lanh knew that, just like her mother, she had contracted the hepatitis B virus as an infant, while still in Vietnam, but she'd always enjoyed robust health. Her family doctor didn't seem to think she had anything to fear, because she had no signs that the virus was still active. For a second opinion, she sought out a gastroenterologist who was listed in the "top doctors," since gastroenterology includes the liver. This doctor did a blood test and reassured her not to worry. Eighteen months later, Lanh was reaching across the seat of her minivan when she felt a searing pain under her rib cage on the right side. At the emergency room, they found a grapefruit-size cancer in her liver. She found out, too late, that Asians like her who contract hepatitis B in infancy have a huge risk of developing liver cancer in middle age, and that a true liver specialist would have done a different test, an ultrasound of the liver, that likely would have found the cancer while it was still small and curable. Lanh went to a top surgeon at Sloan Kettering in New York, who took out half her liver and thought at first that he'd removed all of the cancer, but it came back three years later, and she died at age forty. Like so many of my other clients, she felt disbelief and betrayal that the gastroenterologist knew so much less about the hepatitis virus than she assumed. Lanh's story is a sad one, but the lesson is clear: Whenever you discover that you have an unusual condition, always seek out a specialist who regularly works with people just like you. Lanh's "top doctor" thought he knew enough about hepatitis because he had dealt with it in patients who had contracted the virus as adults, when the disease is usually mild. That's a completely different situation from a baby whose liver fills with the virus because their immune system hasn't yet matured and who then lives with the virus for decades. Lanh could have found out that she was different only by close questioning and research. It really wasn't her fault; she trusted her top-notch doctor. But that's not enough; you have to be more vigilant.

Looking Up Doctors' Discipline and Lawsuit Records

In every state, you can check with the licensing board for lawsuits and disciplinary actions against a doctor you may be considering. The

Federation of State Medical Boards provides a list of the state medical boards at http://www.fsmb.org. Public Citizen's Health Research Group puts out a ranking of the licensing boards by how many licensing actions they take per year per 1,000 doctors. In the most recent rankings, the range was from 1.18 actions per 1,000 physicians in South Carolina to 8.33 in Alaska, a sevenfold difference.[2] This list can help you judge how aggressive or lax your own state board is, but again, it's not a guarantee of good medicine even if you live in an aggressive state.

You can pay for a search by a company like HealthGrades (http://www.healthgrades.com); this unfortunately will give you little more than what is already out there in the public domain. You can also check other consumers' experiences at Angieslist.com; the views of other consumers will give you good insight into a prospective doctor's people skills, but won't guarantee how truly knowledgeable and insightful that doctor is. The fact is that there is no good, simple rating system for doctors. You have to ask the hard questions and experience the doctor's care, as we discussed in Chapter 5, to find out for yourself.

Lifesavers:

Finding the Best Takes a Lot More Than Avoiding the Worst

You can check medical discipline and malpractice lawsuits on the Web sites mentioned in this chapter. However, this will not tell you much about whether a doctor is right for you. The harder but more necessary work is to go through the steps in Chapter 5 to look for a primary-care doctor whose skills match your specific needs and who is a good listener and diagnostician.

7

Drugs: A Dose of Reality About the Prescription Drug Industry and How You Can Safely Use Medicines

To manage your medicines sensibly, you need to know a lot more than what their names are and when to swallow them. First, you need a dose of the political and social reality of prescription drugs in America. My next prescription is to show you a little about the use and abuse of statistics in medicine, and how numbers are manipulated to support supposed drug "breakthroughs." Finally we will work through a checklist of the key practical advice for safe and sensible use of medicines.

> *Step Four:*
> **Learn the safe, sensible—and skeptical—approach to using medicines.**

Have you ever noticed the pharmaceutical industry's tentacles in your doctor's office? Pick up the pen to sign in on arrival; it likely has the name of some new prescription drug running down the side. Or look at the sticky notepads, the prescription pads, the preprinted forms for medical records. Every little thing is branded with drug logos. Ever seen an attractive, well-dressed young woman lugging a fat, square briefcase down the hall of the doctors' suite? She's not a doctor, not even a nurse. She probably has, at most, six weeks of training on the drugs she is promoting. Your doctor may be relying on her, and her myriad freebies, to make important decisions about what drugs, and how many drugs, you receive. Worse is what you cannot see in your doctor's office. The thought leaders of American medicine, who teach frontline doctors the latest developments in prescription drugs and medical devices, often turn out to be in the pockets of the drug and device manufacturers. Through "lecture fees," "honoraria," "consulting fees," and other payments that can exceed $1 million in only a few years for a well-placed opinion leader, the manufacturers turn medical-school department chairmen and other leaders from neutral experts into propaganda machines.[1]

Americans spend more on drugs per person than anywhere else on the planet. And we are not healthier for it. In fact, we suffer huge numbers of unnecessary injuries from drugs. The numbers stagger the mind:

- Every year, 3.4 billion prescriptions are filled in retail pharmacies and by mail order in the United States. The average is twenty-four prescriptions per year for every man and woman over age sixty-five, and ten per year for those younger than sixty-five.
- Two million Americans are seriously hurt by adverse reactions to drugs every year, and 100,000 of those are fatal injuries.
- The U.S. Food and Drug Administration approves about twenty-five new drugs each year for prescription use, but a significant number of those will eventually be removed from the market or have their usage curtailed because of injuries and death.

You can do a lot to reduce the risk that you or a loved one—and elderly Americans are especially vulnerable—will be hurt by a drug that was meant to help. This chapter will show you how to be appropriately skeptical and cautious about taking medications, and how to do the best with the medications that you do take.

What You Must Know About Drugs and the FDA

The top three editors of the *New England Journal of Medicine*, widely acknowledged as the leading medical research journal in the world, wrote about the FDA in an editorial in 2008: "Owing in part to a lack of resources, approval of a new drug by the FDA is not a guarantee of its safety. . . . FDA approval is usually based on short-term efficacy studies, not long-term safety studies. Despite the diligent attention of the FDA, serious safety issues often come to light only after a drug has entered the market. The FDA, which—unlike most other federal agencies—has no subpoena power, knows only what manufacturers reveal."[2]

And what about those manufacturers? You can learn a lot just from the titles of recent books by responsible health-care authorities. For example, Dr. Marcia Angell, a former top editor at the *New England Journal of Medicine*, wrote a book called *The Truth About the Drug Companies: How They Deceive Us and What to Do About It.*[3] Or look at Shannon Brownlee's book *Overtreated: Why Too Much Medicine Is Making Us Sicker and Poorer;*[4] her chapter on how the drug industry promotes to doctors is titled "Money, Drugs, and Lies." Countless other books and studies have documented how, from the Vioxx scandal to the fen-phen scandal, the drug industry has withheld important safety information, oversold the benefits of its products, and flexed the political muscle that comes with $700 billion in annual revenues to keep regulatory agencies like the FDA at bay.

Health-care insiders know that the studies used to win FDA approval for a new drug barely scratch the surface of the drug's eventual safety profile. Think about it: You take, at most, 5,000 volunteers, make sure they're all healthy before they join the study, and then give them the drug for a maximum of a few months. If no huge problems develop in the volunteers, and if the drug seems to work at least as well as competitors already on the market, that's about all a drug company needs to win approval. Then the drug is released onto the market, and suddenly, once the manufacturer cranks up its marketing machine, hundreds of thousands, even millions of patients are taking the drug, some for years. And many of them are people who were deliberately kept out of the preapproval studies: pregnant women, elderly people, children, anyone with some other health problem besides the one being studied. In effect, the early years that a drug is sold to the public are just a continuation of the experiments that brought the drug to market. Except now the experiment lacks any systematic collection of data on the participants and oversight by safety regulators. Because another scandal of the drug industry is that manufacturers, except in special cases, aren't required to keep track of who gets their drugs or how those people fare once the drug is approved for general use. All that the manufacturers have to do is report to the FDA any adverse reactions that come to their attention, but hospitals and doctors have no requirement to make such reports. So a lot of the millions of adverse reactions that happen every year never are reported to anyone.

Even the preapproval studies aren't free of bias. You may be shocked to discover the percentage of the new drugs approved for use in the United States that are put to independent tests, tests not sponsored by the manufacturer of the drug, before the FDA puts on its stamp of approval:

Zero percent.

A lot of people assume the FDA does its own tests on drugs before they reach the market. In fact, the government relies totally on manufacturers to run the tests and to honestly report the results. (One recent innovation, a baby step in the right direction, promises to end the old practice of manufacturers deep-sixing the results of any study that didn't come out the right way. Now there will be a central registry of all drug studies, so that independent experts can have all the facts when they compare drugs to figure out which are safest and most effective.)

Unpaid Guinea Pigs

Here's the bottom line about new drugs: Unless you feel good about being an unpaid guinea pig, you should avoid any drug in its first few years on the market. The only exception should be for a genuine breakthrough drug that offers treatment for some condition that was untreatable before. Very few of the new drugs that come on the market each year are breakthroughs; most are me-too drugs, designed to grab some of the market share from the most lucrative moneymakers already sold.

This advice goes against the grain of what the advertising industry drills into us consumers: This year's model is always better than last year's. Even when we think we're too smart to fall for that, our credit-card statements often prove otherwise. And with medicines, many of us are disappointed if our personal doctor doesn't hand out free bubble-pack samples of the latest new drugs. *What's wrong with him? Doesn't he keep up?* The truth, that wise and excellent doctors are skeptical about new drugs, is so counterintuitive that you may want to read this twice to make sure it sinks in.

How long should you wait? Dr. Sidney Wolfe, a drug-industry scourge who founded Public Citizen's Health Research Group three decades ago, has a seven-year rule. He based this on a look-back study of 548 drugs approved over twenty-five years by the FDA; they found a one in five chance that the drug would either be required to put a major new warning on its label (called a black-box warning because it appears in a black-bordered box at the top of the professional label) or would be ordered off the market. Half of the new black-box warnings happened within the first seven years of use, and half of the removals from market happened in the first two years. Vioxx was on the market six years before its removal due to the risk of heart attacks. The *fen* part of *fen-phen*—officially called dexfenfluramine and branded Pondimin or Redux—was on the market for eighteen months before its removal due to life-threatening lung and heart-valve toxicity.

One encouraging sign for the future is an emerging consensus that independent studies of drugs need to be done to produce the best evidence for what drugs work and what don't. The model for this was a study, funded by the U.S. Congress, called the Women's Health Initiative (WHI), which started in 1991 and eventually enrolled some 160,000 volunteers, all postmenopausal women in generally good health. The WHI was supervised by the National Heart, Lung, and Blood Institute, part of the National Institutes of Health in Bethesda, Maryland. In 2001 the WHI published a series of landmark reports that proved hormone "replacement" therapy for menopausal women (that clever little word *replacement* helped subtly sell the naturalness of the whole concept) did not help prevent heart attacks and was not good for Alzheimer's. In fact, the government researchers showed, giving estrogens to women at menopause actually can cause heart attack, stroke, and breast cancer. Before this report, Wyeth, Pfizer, and other big drug companies made billions of dollars with aggressive campaigns that promoted their estrogen drugs for daily use by virtually every older woman. After all, who doesn't want to cut their risk of heart attack and stay healthy? Actress Lauren Hutton offered her gap-toothed smile on television ads for Wyeth's Prempro. All these ads would end with the tagline, "Ask your doctor." What consumers didn't know was that their doctors were also subject to a marketing blitz by sales reps who visited as often as every week. Now, if you ask your doctor what influence the free stuff—especially the free samples in the bubble packs—has on her prescription writing, you will be told, "Absolutely none." And she might add, "No one can buy me off for a free lunch." Except that the manufacturers know better. They subscribe to databases sold by marketing companies that are wired into every retail pharmacy in America. The pharmacies transmit prescription information to a central computer every day; the only thing stripped out is the patient's name. Sales reps download weekly, even daily reports that tell them exactly how much bang they get for the buck with every doctor on their sales routes. So they quickly learn who responds to free lunches, and who might need a little extra, say a dinner or a free trip. And they know a secret: Virtually everybody who accepts gifts, even small ones, changes their prescribing habits. It's just human nature. Psychologists have a name for it: the reciprocity instinct.

Prescription for Good Doctors: No Free Lunch

The good news is that some doctors and big medical institutions are rebelling. Bob Goodman, a Brooklyn, New York, internist, started a group called No Free Lunch. If you go to its Web site, http://www.nofreelunch.org, you'll find items like the Pen Amnesty, where doctors can send in their free pens emblazoned with drug names and in return receive pens that say PharmFree. And doctors can get a suitable-for-framing certificate if they take the "pledge," which says, "I, ______, am committed to practicing medicine in the best interest of my patients and on the basis of the best available evidence, rather than on the basis of advertising or promotion. I therefore pledge to accept no money, gifts, or hospitality from the pharmaceutical industry; to seek unbiased sources of information and not rely on information disseminated by drug companies; and to avoid conflicts of interest in my practice, teaching, and/or research." You can search the No Free Lunch Web site for doctors who've taken the pledge, although so far, only a handful are listed.[5]

Leading medical schools like Stanford have recognized the problem and now ban pharmaceutical freebies from campus. The American Medical Student Association also has an active PharmFree program. As young medical graduates come into practice in the next few years, you can expect to see new doctors showing a more skeptical, "just the facts, ma'am" approach to evidence justifying the use of the latest and greatest pharmaceutical drugs. In the meantime, here is some information to arm you for your own reading of the evidence.

Understanding the Hyped Numbers Behind the New Studies

Wednesday is breakthrough day if you watch television news. That's publication day for some of the top weekly American medical journals, like the *New England Journal of Medicine.* Nearly every week, some new study on prescription drugs hits the airwaves as a "breakthrough." Pages of dense medical prose are distilled down to one or two arresting numbers, like "50 percent improvement in . . ." or "20 percent fewer . . . ." Don't count on your doctor to go back and read the original article with a skeptical eye and pick up on all the caveats that cut these numbers down to a less impressive size. He has seen the PowerPoint from the drug manufacturer's sales rep, and the drug sounds wonderful. But is it really?

Let's do a case study on one of the last big "breakthroughs" before this book went to press: The headline said that statin drugs for lowering cholesterol had been proven to cut heart attacks by 50 percent in some patients who already had normal cholesterol levels. So that means everybody should take a statin, right? It's the new multivitamin. And sure enough, within twenty-four hours of publication in late 2008, medical leaders were saying that millions of Americans (on top of the millions with actual high cholesterol already taking statins) would now be written prescriptions for these drugs, on the assumption that the 50 percent benefit in heart attacks would far outweigh the risks and side effects and costs of the drugs.

So what is behind this "50 percent" number?

The study tested people who were put on cholesterol-lowering statins because they had an abnormally high result on a blood test called C-reactive protein, even though the same people did not have high cholesterol. C-reactive protein (CRP for short) is a marker for inflammation in the blood vessels, and inflammation is thought to be a prime reason why arteries feeding the heart become blocked and the patient suffers a heart attack. So it was a natural hypothesis to test.

Half the patients in the study swallowed the statin drug, and the other half, assigned by a coin flip, took a sugar pill, a placebo, instead. That's the standard "randomized" way to run a drug-efficacy study; it cuts out the potential for bias when one of the comparison groups might turn out to be healthier than the other. So far so good.

The first hint of a major caveat for the study's results is the large number of volunteers who were kicked out of the study before it even started. The researchers recruited 90,000 volunteers but rejected eight in ten of them because they had arthritis, some other kind of inflammation, or another condition that the researchers thought might interfere with the results. They ended up selecting 17,802 participants for the study.[6] Why does this make for a red flag on the study's applicability? Because in the real world, there are plenty of people like the volunteers who were rejected, and they are going to be offered this drug now by doctors who haven't read the fine print of the study to see that this kind of patient wasn't even tested.

But let's leave that aside and go on to look at the actual headline number: the 50 percent reduction in heart attacks. What does it mean? As I explain in more detail in Chapter 8, you can never understand what any medical statistic really means unless you translate it into actual numbers of real people. You will hear this several times from me: Count the people if you want the truth. In the statin-CRP study, here is how the numbers shake out.

In the placebo group, 18 of every 1,000 patients suffered a heart attack or some other serious heart event during the study. In the group taking the statin drug, 9 of every 1,000 patients had a serious heart event. That's how the researchers could report that the risk had been cut in half—from 18 to 9—although the actual numbers of patients were few. Comparing 18 to 9 is called a relative-risk ratio; these numbers tend to be more impressive and thus are favored by the drug manufacturer marketing machines. Comparing 18 in 1,000 to 9 in 1,000 is called comparing the absolute risk. The absolute-risk number is a real-world number that tells consumers what we need to know. In this case, it means that only 1 percent of the study participants—9 in 1,000, or about 1 in 100—avoided a heart attack by taking the statin drug.

Another important number for patients to understand, in figuring out if a new medicine is for them, is called the "number needed to treat." How many patients need to be treated with the new drug for one patient to benefit? According to a *New England Journal of Medicine* editorial, which analyzed the statin-CRP study, *120* patients would need to be treated with statins over two years for just *1* of those patients to benefit.

That number might be enough to persuade some patients to take the drug. But it's a lot different than 50 percent. Bottom line: To make intelligent choices about treatments, patients need to understand how many patients like them are really expected to benefit from the treatment. You can learn these answers by focusing on how many actual people are helped by the treatment. Do not focus on misleading, vague numbers like "50 percent improvement." Fifty percent of what? Focusing on real numbers of real people will give you the answer.

Now, I don't expect every reader to pour through the fine print of the *New England Journal of Medicine* and do independent evaluations of drug studies. I do expect you to be appropriately skeptical about "breakthroughs" after you've read this chapter. And there is a lot you can do to protect yourself just by knowing that (1) numbers are easily manipulated but (2) it's not that hard to find the kernel of truth behind a medical statistic if you make sure to count the number of patients. We will return to this "count the people" approach to understanding medical statistics twice more in this book: when we talk about what you need to know about medical testing error rates in Chapter 8 and when we go over cancer-survival numbers in Chapter 15.

Essentials for the Safe Use of Drugs

So whom do you trust? Personally, I look to independent-minded primary-care doctors who don't accept a boatload of freebies from the drug reps. Some forward-thinking HMOs like Kaiser Permanente also bar pharmaceutical gifts and do their own evaluations of what drugs are appropriate for their patients. And I look to independent Web sites like Public Citizen's Health Research Group (http://www.citizen.org/hrg/) and the Medical Letter (http://www.medicalletter.org), which has been publishing independent no-holds-barred reviews of drugs since 1959. It accepts no advertising and relies entirely on subscription revenue for its critical appraisals of new drugs and for its recommendations based on expert consensus.

Here are some questions to ask yourself to improve your personal drug safety. If you have an elderly parent, consider answering these questions for them too.

1. ***How many drugs are you taking?*** An enormous problem, especially for older Americans, is taking too many drugs at one time, because these drugs can have dangerous interactions with each other or with other things you consume like alcohol, caffeine, and grapefruit juice. (Yes, grapefruit juice. It powerfully alters the way that the liver processes many drugs and generally should not be taken by anyone who has to use prescription drugs every day, unless your doctor or pharmacist says it's okay.)

2. ***Do you have an up-to-date list of all your medications?*** I've already talked briefly in Chapter 2 about making and keeping an up-to-date list of all the medications you take. That's why you should always use the same pharmacy if you can, because its computer can automatically flag possible bad interactions among the prescriptions you've had filled there. This list of medications is so important that Dr. Sidney Wolfe makes it his first rule on his list of ten rules for safer drug use.[7] He calls it having a "brown-bag session" with your primary doctor. You throw all your pill bottles in a brown bag—and don't forget over-the-counter drugs and dietary supplements, anything you take regularly—and take them to the doctor's office. Then, together, you fill out a drug worksheet that lists every drug, how and when you take it, what for, and problems to watch out for. You can also do this

with your pharmacist. A blank form to get you started can be pulled from Public Citizen's Web site.[8]

3. ***Do you really need all those medications?*** The next step in safer drug use is to make sure you need all those drugs in your brown bag. Mildly high blood pressure, anxiety, mild adult-onset diabetes, and constipation are some of the most notorious ailments that lead to overuse of drugs. Eating right, exercising daily, and other good health habits can eliminate the need for a lot of these. Also, a drug might have helped you for a few months, but maybe you no longer need it. That's why regular review of all your drugs with your doctor is important. Obviously, you need a doctor's advice before you throw away any pills.

4. ***Are you candid with your doctor?*** If a drug doesn't seem to work or it causes some strange new symptom, a lot of people will stop taking the drug without telling the doctor, sometimes out of a misplaced fear of hurting the doctor's feelings. As with every other aspect of health care, total honesty is the only way to win good care.

5. ***Have you had a bad reaction to a new medication?*** One other thing you should know is to keep your antennae up for a bad reaction, especially in the first few weeks you're on a new drug. It's a good idea to assume that any new symptom you develop after starting a new drug might be caused by that drug, and you should call the doctor immediately. Some adverse drug reactions can be nipped in the bud this way. One especially tragic reaction that I've seen several times in clients is tardive dyskinesia: permanent, uncontrollable shaking and other movements in the face, arms, or legs. Another is an allergic burn of the skin and mucous membranes (lips, nostrils, eyelids, etc.), called Stevens-Johnson syndrome, which can be fatal if it goes too far.

Some bad reactions to drugs can be subtle, especially in older people. Many of us assume that Grandpa's mind is getting foggy because of old age, when it really might be from the fistful of drugs he swallows every day. Depression can also be caused by drugs. The best gift you might give an elderly parent who seems to be "losing it" could be to take them to an appointment with a doctor who specializes in geriatrics for a comprehensive drug review.

Lifesavers:

The Step-Four Checklist for Healthy Medication Management

1. Avoid new prescription drugs until they've been on the market for at least two years, and better, seven years.
2. Unless you have a unique and rare condition, you're usually better off with tried-and-true drugs that have been on the market for a long time. All generics fit this bill because the brand-name drug's patent has expired. Generics are also a lot cheaper. I'm no fan of insurance companies, but often, if they hassle your doctor and resist paying for a new drug she wants to prescribe for you, there may be a good reason: The old tried-and-true drug might be safer and better for you.
3. Try to find a primary-care doctor who doesn't accept gifts from the drug manufacturers and who gets his drug education from independent sources like *the Medical Letter on Drugs and Therapeutics.*
4. Make a worksheet of all the drugs you're taking. If you have an elderly relative who cannot do this for themselves, it's especially important for you to step in and help. Pull a blank form from Public Citizen's Web site, or ask your pharmacist or primary-care doctor to help.
5. Review your drug worksheet with your primary-care doctor on a regular basis. Look for ways you can safely reduce the number of drugs and the size of the dosages. Healthy habits like diet and exercise are sometimes the best substitute for a drug, especially when you have some kind of borderline abnormality.

continues

6. When you start a new drug, assume that any new symptom you develop in the first few weeks is coming from the drug, and call your doctor promptly.
7. Always be totally candid and frank with your primary-care doctor about all the drugs you're taking, whether they're prescribed by this doctor or someone else, and don't forget the over-the-counter drugs, diet supplements, alcohol, and caffeine that you take in.
8. Check the following sources for unbiased drug information:

Public Citizen Health Research Group at http://www.worstpills.org;

Medical Letter at http://www.medicalletter.org;

Therapeutics Letter (Canada)—established in 1994 by the Department of Pharmacology and Therapeutics at the University of British Columbia "to provide physicians and pharmacists with up to date, evidence-based, practical information on rational drug therapy," at http://www.ti.ubc.ca;

Drug and Therapeutics Bulletin (U.K.)—a monthly publication giving independent evaluations of and practical advice on individual treatments and the management of disease, at http://www.dtb.org.uk; and

Prescriber's Letter at http://www.prescribersletter.com.

8

"Should I Be Tested?" Why Understanding the Numbers Is Crucial

> *Step Five:*
> **Understand why all medical tests are flawed, and seek a second or third opinion at every major crossroads of health care.**

Nearly every day, somewhere in the United States, a woman in her mid-forties undergoes a mammogram and is later told she has tested "positive" for a suspicious mass. How worried should she be? What should she do next? This chapter explores why, to be a smart consumer of health care, you need to understand a little about medical statistics. Every single decision in medicine—to test, to treat, to watch and wait—is based at least in part on statistical evidence—evidence that both doctors and patients regularly misunderstand. Needless heartache is but one of the consequences of our numerical illiteracy. In this and the next chapter, I will show you that all tests have built-in error, and therefore you should never let a single test result dictate an important medical decision. That's why Step Five on my list of the Necessary Nine steps is, "Understand why all tests are flawed, and seek a second or third opinion at every major crossroads of health care."

In Chapter 7, we saw, in the study of patients who were tested for C-reactive protein, how a supposed 50 percent reduction in heart attack from use of statins shrank to a mere 1 percent reduction when we counted the actual number of people helped by the drug. The same kind of technique—counting actual numbers of people instead of confusing percentages—will help us to understand the meaning of a positive mammogram for a patient in her midforties.

Let's eavesdrop on a conversation between doctor and patient after a positive mammogram:

PATIENT: "So this means I have cancer? I need a mastectomy?"

DOCTOR: "It's not 100 percent. But mammograms do have a 90 percent accuracy rate."

PATIENT: "You're saying chances are nine out of ten that I have cancer?"

DOCTOR: "What the number means is that nine out of ten women who actually have cancer will test positive on a mammogram. And if they don't have cancer, there is an even higher accuracy rate, about 93 percent, which means a 7 percent false-alarm rate."

PATIENT: "You're confusing me with a lot of numbers. It still sounds like it's highly likely that I have cancer and that I'm going to need surgery."

DOCTOR: "You will need further testing, but I'm afraid that's right."

The truth is that both doctor and patient are confused. If we count the people, we can sort out the surprising truth: A 90 percent accurate medical test can actually be 90 percent wrong. This counting technique works for any medical test, and it helps sort out basic questions of whether you should have a test in the first place and what it means when the test comes out one way or the other.

I have adapted this example from a brilliant book by a German statistics professor, Gerd Gigerenzer, *Calculated Risks*.[1] His key insight is that true risks can best be calculated by counting actual numbers of people instead of using percentages, which can be vague, confusing, and highly misleading.

From Confusion to Clarity: Count Real People

We need to plug in one additional number to understand the meaning of a positive mammogram test for a woman in her forties: the incidence of actual breast cancer in women in their forties. That rate is about 8 in 1,000. So in a group of 1,000 fortyish women, 992 do not have breast cancer, and 8 do. When these women undergo mammograms, 90 percent of those with cancer will test positive, and 93 percent without cancer will test truly negative. That last number also means that 7 percent of women in their forties without cancer will receive a false alarm: a "false positive" test result, as the awkward nomenclature of medical testing has it.

When we count the people, here's how it works out.

- Of the 992 women with no cancer, 7 percent will still receive a positive result, a false positive. That means about 70 (rounded off) will test falsely positive, a false alarm, and the other 922 will test truly negative.
- Of the 8 who do have breast cancer, 90 percent of those, or around 7 of the 8, will test positive, and that will be a "true positive." One will actually have breast cancer but will test negative (a "false negative").
- So in our group of 1,000 women in their forties who've had mammograms, 77 have tested positive—70 who don't have cancer, and 7 who do. The chances that our patient with a positive mammogram really has breast cancer are 7 out of 77, or 9 percent. That's a ways off from 90 percent!

This figure shows visually what the preceding paragraphs have explained:

Figure 1: What does it mean when the mammogram tests "positive"?

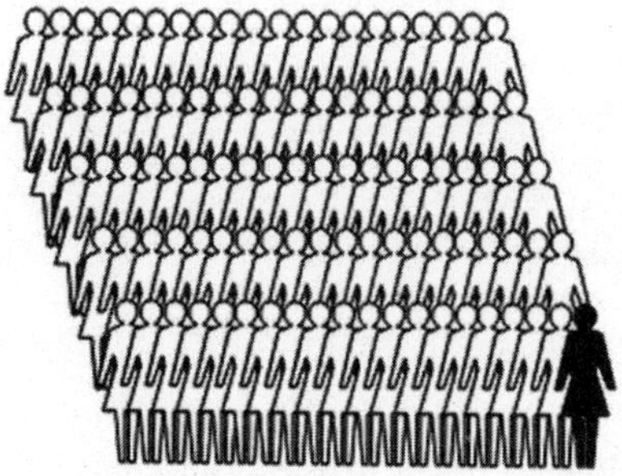

A. Fewer than one in one hundred women in their forties have breast cancer. If everyone undergoes mammogram, and the mammogram has a 90% accuracy rate, here is the result:

B. The one woman with actual cancer will test positive nine out of ten times.

C. When the other ninety-nine women without cancer are tested, they have a one in ten chance of testing false positive. So testing all one hundred women will result in ten positives: one true positive and nine false positives.

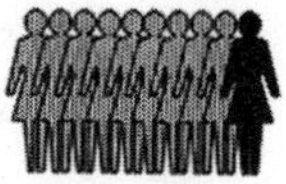

D. So a "positive" mammogram result on a woman in her forties only has only a ten percent chance of being correct, even when the test is 90% accurate.

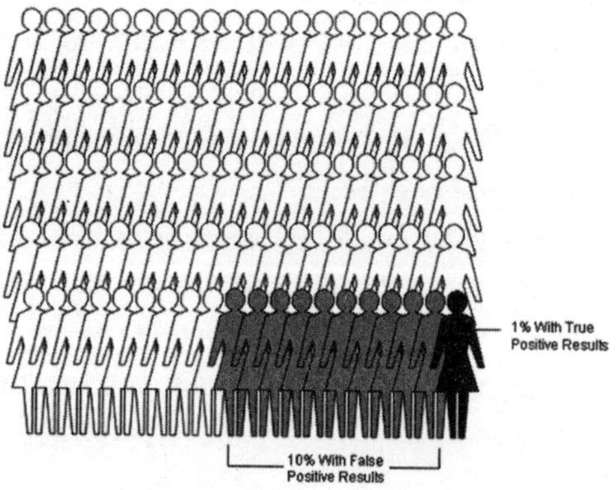

This is true for every kind of medical test, from sophisticated brain MRI scans to the humble urine test; no medical test is perfectly accurate. Every medical test has an error rate—actually every test has two error rates: overcounting and undercounting the number of people who actually have the disease. When overcounting happens, false alarms are raised. The test seems to show you have breast cancer, but further tests prove you do not. Patients who don't understand this, and who go straight to surgery without confirmatory tests, undergo unnecessary breast removals. As we have just seen with women in their forties getting mammograms, false positives are a big problem whenever the number of people in the test population who actually have the disease is very low, because many patients undergo needless anxiety and expensive tests for nothing.

The opposite kind of error is undercounting the number of people with disease. When undercounting happens, patients are falsely reassured; this type of error is called a false negative. The test seems to give a clean bill of health, but only because it has missed the disease that is really there. False negatives (as we will see below) are a big problem whenever the incidence of the disease in the population being studied is very high, because many patients miss out on treatment they need. (See the endnote for a few more terms you will often hear when doctors talk about the statistics of testing.[2])

Another example shows how understanding the numbers can be a matter of life and death. When AIDS testing first became widespread in the mid-1980s, a combination of two tests was used to confirm if the test subject had AIDS. Some people with "confirmed" AIDS, who were told that the error rate of the combination test was only 1 in 10,000, were so distraught they committed suicide. Many of these victims did not have AIDS; neither the patients nor their doctors understood that all it takes is a tiny false-positive error rate in a test being conducted in a low-risk population to produce as many false alarms as accurate results. When we count the people, we can easily see why. In a group of 10,000 men without risk factors for AIDS (intravenous drug use, unprotected homosexual activity, etc.), only 1 in the 10,000 actually has AIDS.[3] The test for AIDS (a two-part test on the same blood sample, called ELISA and Western Blot) is 99.9 percent accurate (i.e., it has a 0.1 percent false-negative rate) for those who have the disease, and it generates false-positive results only 0.01 percent of the time. So what does that mean when a man in this low-risk population tests positive? The one man who actually has AIDS in this group will very likely test positive, but another man without AIDS will also test positive, because 0.01 percent false positive translates into a 1 in 10,000 false-positive rate. So among every 10,000 low-risk men, 2 of the men test positive, but only 1 has AIDS. The odds are 1 in 2, not 999 out of 1,000 (the same as 99.9 percent) and not 9,999 out of 10,000 (the same as 99.99 percent). The false-alarm problem is even worse if the test has an accuracy rate of 99 percent. In the same group of 10,000 people, only 1 of whom actually has the disease, 100 will test false positive (1 percent of 10,000). So a 99 percent accurate test can produce a positive test that is 99 percent likely to be wrong![4]

Now, if the same test with the same accuracy is administered to a high-risk population, the proportion that will test falsely positive is much lower. In a group of homosexual men, the proportion with AIDS will be on the order of 150 in 10,000. Of those, nearly all of the 150 (99.9 percent) will test positive, and of the remaining uninfected men who are tested, only 1 of the 9,850 will test false positive without having the disease (remember the false-positive rate is 1 in 10,000). So of the 151 men who test positive, 150 have the disease and only 1 does not. So the false-positive problem goes away if the test population is at high risk.

This shows that false alarms are a big problem when low-risk populations are tested. If a high-risk population is tested, the problem is false reassurance from false-negative results. Let's run through another hypothetical example: MRI imaging of the knee for someone who developed sudden, sharp knee pain with exercise, and the pain hasn't gone away after a few days of ice and taking it easy. Eighty percent of those people (I'm making up this percentage just to make a point) will turn out to have torn cartilage or ligament in the knee that needs surgery. Now assume the MRI machine has a 10 percent false-positive rate and a 10 percent false-negative rate. So you're the patient. After a week of terrible knee pain, you have hobbled into the radiology office for an MRI. Afterwards, you're told the test came out negative. Should you accept that or ask for a second opinion or a second test? In other words, what are the chances it was a false negative? Let's work through the numbers using Professor Gigerenzer's approach. Of 100 people like you, 80 actually have a torn cartilage or torn ligament. Of those 80, 8 will test false negative (a 10 percent false-negative rate). Of the 20 without any tear, only 2 will test false positive (a 10 percent false-positive rate), so 18 will test truly negative. So we add up the total negative tests: 8 false negatives plus 18 true negatives, 26 total. That means that your chance of being falsely negative is 8 out of 26, or about 30 percent.

Notice how straightforward the calculation is when we count actual people, and how hard the calculation is when we think about percentages. ("Let's see, I have an 80 percent chance of having a tear inside my knee, but the MRI doesn't see anything, and the MRI is 90 percent accurate. So now what?") Most of us would throw up our hands at that point; we would have absolutely no idea how to calculate our chances of being in the false-reassurance group—just like most women who are told their mammogram tested "positive" have no idea how to determine their odds of being in the false-alarm group.

If you think that improved technology will make this discussion outdated, think again. Any statistician will tell you that false-positive and false-negative rates are on a seesaw with each other. You can make one go down, but that makes the other go up. This happens regularly with new imaging technology that lets us see ever-finer detail in breast, brain, and other important parts of the body. What that exquisite level of detail does is drive down the false negative rate—because we see more, there is a lower chance of missing something. But when we see more, we see a lot of blips that look wrong but turn out not to be anything—that is, the false-positive rate goes up.

More Eye-Opening Numbers: The Risk in Not Understanding Benefit Versus Risk

We've talked about the risk of medical tests being wrong. Now let's focus on the other side of the coin: the benefit of the test being right. Numbers about the benefits of tests and treatments are thrown around all the time, often to misleading effect, as we already saw in Chapter 7 about the statin study and C-reactive protein. What about the potential benefits of breast-cancer screening? This is a different set of numbers than the ones we've just discussed about the risks of the test being wrong. We will see again that numbers are used in misleading ways, and on the plus side, the solution I advocate is the same simple one as before: Count the actual numbers of patients in the different categories, and let patients judge for themselves the real benefits.

Many women have heard that if they're over forty, they can cut their chances of dying from breast cancer by 25 percent by getting an annual mammogram. So because they also know that women have a one in ten chance of getting breast cancer, they steel themselves and go through the screening, or they put off the test but in the meantime feel scared and guilty. What is wrong with this picture? Plenty. Let's start with the 1-in-10 number, which has terrorized so many women. What does it really mean? Let's translate it into actual numbers of real people: If you take any group of 1,000 women and follow them over their lifetimes, by the time they reach age eighty-five, roughly 99 of them, or 1 in 10, will have developed breast cancer.[5] A handful will be diagnosed with breast cancer in their thirties, a few more in their forties, still a few more in their fifties, and so on, until eventually, a total of 99 of the 1,000, or 1 in 10, will develop breast cancer. And only a fraction of these will actually die of breast cancer. In the meantime, many more will have died of other causes. But many women who hear the 1 in 10 number think that it applies no matter how old they are, and so women in their forties are petrified at the idea that they have a 1 in 10 chance of getting breast cancer in the next few years. That's a wild overestimate. For the average woman without special risk factors, the chances of developing cancer in her forties are more like 8 in 1,000, as we discussed earlier in this chapter.

Another way to use actual numbers of people to win some perspective on the potential benefits of screening is to tally the number of deaths every year. According to the National Institutes of Health, 40,000 American women die of breast cancer each year, but in the same year 329,000 die of heart diseases, 87,000 from stroke, 73,000 from lung cancer, and 68,000 from noncancerous obstructive lung disease.[6] So a healthy respect for breast cancer is appropriate, but it doesn't deserve to be the most-feared disease for American women when eight times more of them die of heart disease each year and nearly twice as many die of lung cancer.

What about saving lives with screening tests intended to catch early cancers? Here is how that statistic of a 25 percent reduction in deaths translates in the real world. If you thought that means that of every 100 women screened, 25 of them would be saved by mammograms, you would be making a natural assumption that many others have made, but you would be very far off the mark. The actual numbers come from a series of studies in Sweden involving some 280,000 women. Of those over age forty who did not undergo mammograms, 4 in 1,000 died of breast cancer over the ten years of the study. Of those over age forty who did have mammograms, 3 in 1,000 died of breast cancer over the same ten years. The reduction from 4 to 3 per 1,000 is where the 25 percent number comes from. Put another way, for every 1,000 women who participate in mammogram screening for ten years, 1 of them will be saved from dying of breast cancer.[7] The odds of saving 1 life are a little improved if screening begins only at age fifty instead of forty. Of every 270 women who start screening mammograms at age fifty and undergo one every other year for the next twenty years, 1 life will be saved—or about 4 in 1,000, which is a lot more than the 1 in 1,000 lives saved for starting mammograms at age forty.

Are those kinds of odds worth it to undergo the trouble of regular screening? That is a personal decision. My only point is that to make that decision rationally and realistically, you need to look at the numbers with eyes wide open.

Lifesavers:

How Understanding Numbers Helps Us Make Better Decisions

I've tried to give you in a few pages a taste of what Professor Gigerenzer teaches in an entire book. I recommend strongly that you read his book, which has many other insights into medical statistics and which he works hard to make easy for math dummies like me. In the meantime, here are the lessons we can draw from this excursion into the numbers behind testing:

- Anytime you're considering a major medical decision based on one test, it's important to remember Ben Franklin's saying, "In this world, nothing is certain but death and taxes." That means you should never let a single test result decide if you have treatment or no treatment. You should at least have a different test, or a repeat test, or another set of eyes looking at the test you've already had. (For more on second opinions, see the next chapter.)
- The accuracy rate of tests can be highly misleading. It all depends on what your risk is going into the test. Low-risk patients need to be wary of the possibility of false alarm test results. High-risk patients need to be wary of the chance of falsely reassuring results. And if there's not enough data out there to know where you fit into the spectrum of risk, you could be facing either or both issues of false alarm or false reassurance.

continues

- If you really want to understand if a test is worthwhile for you, ask the doctor to count the numbers of actual people like you who are benefited from the test and see if that outweighs the number who are hurt by the test.
- Screening tests (undergoing a test without any evidence that you have the disease) make a lot more sense for people who are in high-risk populations. With mammograms, for example, women in their forties who undergo regular screening, without a risk factor like a family background of breast cancer, will have a much higher chance of being scared to death without reason than of early detection of the disease. The older you get, the higher your risk of all kinds of disease, so screening tests start to make more sense. That's why health authorities don't recommend regular screening for adults for most cancers until they are in their fifties. This also means everyone's screening program should be individualized. Women in their forties who do have several risk factors for breast cancer, like the BRCA gene mutation, are good candidates for regular mammograms.[8]
- This discussion also shows why it doesn't make sense to rely on a single negative test result when you're hurting badly and thus are in a high-risk group. Chances are your feelings of pain are right, and the test result is just wrong.
- There is always a trade-off with any new technology. The more sensitive it is at seeing blips inside your body, the more it is going to raise false alarms. On a practical level, that means that if you're young and in good health with no big risk factors for disease (smoking is the biggest), it makes no sense for you to undergo one of those "executive physicals" that puts you through head-to-toe body imaging. The overwhelming likelihood is that it will generate false alarms and a lot of further expensive and dangerous tests that will do you more harm than good.

9

The Second Opinion: Always Your First Choice

We introduced the topic of medical testing and second opinions in Chapter 8 with a focus on the statistics of medical error. Now we will broaden our look at medical tests to consider biopsies, the one test where second looks have been shown over and over to have a dramatic influence on treatment and survival. Then we will consider other circumstances in which second opinions can be very useful. Because insurance companies sometimes hassle you about paying for these second and third opinions, I offer some tips for dealing with insurers. Finally, we will discuss how being alert to your doctor's possible conflicts of interest can push you toward second or third opinions. The goal of all this is to search out the best answers for your unique needs.

Biopsies are one of those tests that everyone has heard of, and so we're too embarrassed to reveal our ignorance by asking exactly what's involved. So here's the scoop. When a surgeon removes anything from just about anywhere in the body, the entire specimen is sent in a tray to the hospital's pathology lab. There it is embedded in wax to preserve it, and samples just a few cells thick are shaved off and mounted on glass slides, just like in high-school biology class. The specimen is stained to highlight anatomic features. Special staining can be done to look for footprints of viruses and other invaders. A pathologist looks at these glass slides under the microscope. If the surgery was for cancer, and the goal was to take out the entire cancer, as it usually is, the pathologist reports back on whether the specimen shows "clean margins," the cancerous cells stopping a healthy distance from the edge of the specimen. Just as important, the pathologist tries to classify the exact kind of cancer and how aggressive it looks.

What laypeople don't often know is that these opinions are fraught with possibility for disagreement and outright error, and that's why getting a second opinion on biopsies—and all other tests, for that matter—is one of the critical nine steps to taking charge of your own health care.

Wallpaper Inspector, Art Critic

I explain to friends that a pathologist's job combines being an inspector in a wallpaper factory with an art critic. The pathologist must inspect the entire specimen, many thousands of cells, that seem to run by forever in repeating swirls and loops under the microscope. The pathologist needs to make sure a specimen that looks completely benign doesn't have any hidden islands of cancer. And once a cancer is spotted, the pathologist's job turns to art critic; he or she has to interpret subtle features of the cells to classify the exact kind of cancer and grade its aggressiveness, all of which makes a big difference in the planning of subsequent treatment. I pick the analogy to art critic for a good reason; you would think that in the study of disease, there are right answers and wrong answers, and everything should be clear-cut. But it's not. Pathologists can debate the diagnosis of a disease with as much passion as art historians debate whether an alleged Jackson Pollock painting is genuine.

Pathologists are important players in the medical-care system, but most patients never meet one. Ironically, they can be very easy to reach on the telephone, since they don't have patients crowding their schedules and thus don't have phalanxes of nurses and secretaries to screen out patients trying to talk to them.

The good news is that a second opinion of a pathology specimen is as close as the nearest Federal Express box, and it's often free or a modest cost. The originating hospital can either send the slides it made to the second-opinion pathologist, or it can shave some "recut" specimens to mail off. Some institutions now do "telemedicine" consultations where the pathologists gather around computer screens to look at digital images of the microscopic specimens.

Sue Carroll's Story

Sue Carroll is a tall woman in her late fifties, with a perky bob of salt-and-pepper hair. Sue bubbles with vigor and cheer, appropriate for her brush with death thirty years ago. Sue is alive today because a coworker at a federal government health agency in Washington, D.C., demanded that she get a second opinion when Sue's surgeon urged a "wait and see" approach as the next step after she'd had surgery for a rare kind of breast cancer.

Sue tells the story best:

> In 1981, I was working at the Department of Health and Human Services, in the Office of Health Information, Health Promotion, Physical Fitness and Sports Medicine (or OHIHPPFSM, pronounced "oh-hip-fizzem"). Prior to that, I'd written a newsletter on public health education, so I was familiar with the world of translating health and medical jargon into more generally accessible information. I was familiar with the concept of being an "activated patient" and a "consumer" of health care.
>
> I was also familiar with breast lumps. I'd had them in various forms since I was fifteen years old. The first one turned out to be a

cyst and just went away on its own, as did most of the others. Four or five of them had been diagnosed as fibroadenomas, a type of benign tumor. Those had been removed by a surgeon at George Washington University Hospital, Dr. Tsangaris—a really nice guy, and one who received at least one award from his students as being a great teacher. How did I find him? I'd worked at GW hospital for a while, and he'd been recommended to me.

When I was fifteen and had the first lump, I assumed it was cancer and that I was going to lose my hair and die. After going through the subsequent string of biopsies and lumpectomies, I'd gotten pretty casual about it. I do remember feeling the 1981 lump (while soaping up in the shower) with concern, and somehow knowing that this one was not a cyst and would probably have to come out. But I wasn't alarmed. It did not occur to me that it would be malignant. I went in to see Dr. Tsangaris; he felt the lump and agreed that it should probably come out, but he was also not overly concerned. So we scheduled the surgery, he took it out, and I went back for the postsurgery checkup a week later ready to dust off the whole incident.

I vividly remember the gray look on his face when he told me the pathologist report said it was a sarcoma. He was shaking his head, saying something about how this couldn't be right, that sarcomas just don't happen in breasts and they certainly don't happen in women as young as I was. (Sarcoma is uncommon: Less than 1 percent of all cancer cases and less than 0.1 percent of breast-cancer cases are sarcomas.) Dr. Tsangaris said, "The pathologist said it was a very low-grade sarcoma. The margins seem to be clean. There's not a high likelihood it will pose a problem. Why don't we just keep our eye on it, and see what happens?"

I rode the bus back to my office, trying to wrap my brain around the idea that this was cancer, and that I was going to have to wait to find out what would happen to me next. It didn't occur to me that there was any option other than doing what my good doctor advised. When I got back to the office, I saw a coworker,

Elaine Bratic, and took her aside to tell her what had just happened. "No!" she said, very firmly. "We are not going to sit back and wait, and we are not going to rely on the word of a pathologist who sees maybe two or three sarcomas a year." Elaine had worked in the Public Affairs office of DHHS for many years, and had contacts all over the agency. She called around, and got me the name of a doctor at the National Institutes of Health who was conducting a study on sarcomas.

I made the next call myself. Would they be interested in reviewing my biopsy slides and giving me a second opinion? The guy on the other end of the phone didn't exactly say, "Way cool!" but he was clearly very interested. It seemed there might be an upside to having a rare cancer.

I retrieved the biopsy slides and report from GW, and took them and myself to NIH. Their pathologist reviewed it all, and determined that (1) it was indeed a sarcoma, and (2) it was of a higher grade—meaning more dangerous—than the GW pathologist had recognized. So they took my case. I had radical surgery, which revealed that the cancer had spread beyond the original tumor. If we had waited "to see what happens" there would have been a recurrence, and quite likely there would have been time for it to spread. And then it would have killed me.

The next couple of years were quite difficult, with extreme radiation treatments, regular bone scans and other nerve-racking tests, more surgeries, and an awful sense of dread. With friends and faith and good work to keep me busy, I got through it. In 1986, the good docs at NIH sent me on my way.

And so here I am, alive and well and happy. I have a lot to be grateful for, and I am, every day. I have spoken to some women's groups about breast cancer, and I tell them there are a few important lessons to take away from my story. One is to know your body—it was really significant that I knew the feel of the lumps in my breast, and knew that this one didn't belong, and would have to come out. Another lesson is to know your doctor—in this case,

I knew him and liked him and could talk to him, but it took Elaine to tell me that this particular doctor didn't know enough about this particular problem to be the one I should listen to. Last but not least, know yourself—know what is important to you and what is not, so that you can nourish yourself through whatever treatment you have to endure, and build a life for yourself that you will fight to hold on to.

Sue was twenty-nine years old when she got the cancer diagnosis. Today, she reports, "I am in great health, happily married, and retired. I am grateful every day to enjoy very pedestrian stuff: cooking, gardening, photography, volunteering at my church, art classes, and (quite literally) dabbling with watercolors. Ray and I like to go camping, and we travel a lot—mostly to visit our children and nine grandchildren who live all around the country. We are also planning our second trip to South Africa, to serve as volunteer instructors at an Anglican seminary in Grahamstown. So I guess it's not all pedestrian. It is all wonderful."

Not So Unusual

If you think Sue's situation is unusual, think again. One study at the University of Michigan Comprehensive Cancer Center found that when breast-cancer patients submitted their biopsy specimens and other records to the UM "tumor board" for a second opinion, fully half of the patients ended up getting some change in their treatment plan.[1]

And it's not limited to breast cancer. Here are some more numbers worth perusing:

- Nearly 1 in 10 pathology cases received a major change in diagnosis leading to significant revisions in treatment and prognosis at Johns Hopkins Hospital.[2]

- A University of Utah Medical School survey found a significant biopsy diagnostic disagreement rate in 2 to 5 of every 100 cases.[3]
- At another institution, a review of pathology cases found major errors in 12 of every 1,000 cases.[4]

These statistics suggest that many thousands of patients have suffered harm from getting either too little or too much treatment because they relied on the first opinion.

Another institution that gives authoritative second opinions on biopsy specimens is the Armed Forces Institute of Pathology, AFIP for short. More people need to know about the AFIP. This Department of Defense agency on the grounds of Walter Reed Army Medical Center, a few miles north of the White House, has 126 pathologists on staff; they provide consultations to doctors all over the world. They have an excellent reputation. Special areas of expertise include:

- skin cancers,
- breast and other female organ cancers,
- genitourinary system,
- liver and other gastrointestinal cancers,
- lung,
- cardiovascular,
- brain and eye, and
- orthopedic pathology.

Turnaround on a consult usually takes a week or less, maybe a bit more if the AFIP is asked to do fancy stuff like electron microscopy (which magnifies what is seen by 100,000 times or more, compared to a few hundred times with a standard microscope).[5] You can contact the AFIP through its Web site: http://www.afip.org.

You can also find Internet-based services that link patients to highly qualified cancer experts. The typical fee is a few hundred dollars, and health insurance will often pay all or most of the charge. One of the most prominent of these services is a group of Harvard-affiliated doctors at three prominent Boston hospitals, Massachusetts General, Brigham & Women's, and the Dana-Farber Cancer Institute. The group calls itself Partners Online Specialty Consultations (https://econsults.partners.org) and provides second opinions for cancer plus other diseases.

Radiology Counts for Second Looks Too

This lesson extends well beyond pathology. In radiology, the accuracy of the images that doctors create of the interior of your body are limited by

- the technical skill of the technician running the test;
- the training and experience of the radiologist interpreting the images; and
- the capacity of the machine to resolve fine detail. Some MRI machines, for example, have much more powerful magnets that show more subtle problems (but that also, as we saw in the last chapter, automatically generate more false alarms).

Most frontline radiologists in typical hospitals are generalists, and there is nothing wrong with that. I have found that a good general radiologist carries around in her head an amazing trove of knowledge about the visual appearance of disease in every part of the body. But there are radiologists who look at nothing but the brain and the spine, or nothing but the chest, or the abdomen, or the bones and joints. NFL players, for example, have their knees imaged about as often as the rest of us get out of bed; do you think the team relies on a general radiologist or a specialist to consult on whether surgery is needed?

All of these radiological subspecialists are available to you; you just have to ask that a specialist be called in. Usually it costs nothing. If one is not on-site, the images can be e-mailed or put on a secure Web site for viewing. The radiology department also can burn a CD of the images that you can view on your home PC or take to another doctor. I have found that a good radiology subspecialist enjoys looking at new and challenging cases; it hones their skills, among other things.

Speaking of on-site, you should be aware that many hospitals now are outsourcing their radiology readings to India or other faraway places, particularly for a scan done outside business hours. Patients are usually blissfully unaware of this; you naturally assume that the person who interprets your scan is in the same building as the scan machine.

Warning Signs for When a New Radiologist Is Really Needed

A radiology second opinion or retest is a good idea if any of the following are true:

- The images are read as "normal" but your body is shrieking to the contrary.
- The report shows uncertainty by the radiologist. This can be evident when the report has a lot of "on the one hand" and "on the other hand" with no firm conclusion. (Sharon Burke's story in Chapter 4 is a good example.)
- The report doesn't address the concerns that led your doctor to ask for the scan.
- The report was issued by a non-subspecialist radiologist.

So with so much at stake and so little expense in improving your odds, here's an easy rule of thumb: If your medical care hinges in any respect on what a pathologist says about what a piece of your body looks like under a microscope, or what a radiologist sees in a picture of your insides, why not put an extra pair of eyes on the case? Especially if that extra pair of eyes has seen hundreds of cases like yours and has made it a life's work to advance the care of people just like you—it's not even a close call, is it?

One more thought: For you to know if your biopsy report or radiology report has red flags and needs another look, you have to dig up and read the report. You don't have to have an MD to tell from a report that a doctor isn't really sure what's wrong with you. You already know how important it is to obtain your own medical records—Step One of our Necessary Nine steps for finding the best health care, for reasons we talked about in Chapter 2. This is just another great reason why you must—must!!!—read what doctors say about your body.

Second Opinions on Surgical Options: Josephine Petrillo's Story

Radiology and pathology reports are only two examples of what qualifies for a second opinion. Here is a story that shows the importance of seeking a second opinion on surgical options. This also introduces the topic of dealing with insurance companies who balk at second opinions or at treatment from someone outside the insurer's list.

Josephine Petrillo is a widow of a bus driver from Staten Island. She is a devout Italian American who walked to Mass every morning for as long as she could. Questioning medical authority is no more in her nature than questioning the Pope. When she was sixty-five, Josephine started noticing that her balance felt slightly off and she could hardly walk in a straight line. It seemed as if her body was pulling her a bit to one side as she walked. At the same time, she sensed some numbness on the right side of her face. For the last several years, her hearing had been worsening in her right ear. After a few visits, her primary care physician ordered an MRI, and an acoustic neuroma was discovered, behind the right ear, pressing into the brain. In hindsight, the four years of gradual hearing loss in her right ear fit exactly with this neuroma; her doctors kept saying it was normal age-related hearing loss without offering any special test, which should have been done since the hearing loss was one-sided. (By the way, it's a good rule of thumb that one-sided symptoms of any kind raise a red flag. The body often distributes real disease, as opposed to normal aging, in an uneven fashion.)

Acoustic neuromas are slow-growing noncancerous tumors of the acoustic nerve, which connects the inner ear to the brain. They usually need to be removed because they can press on important brain structures, but the surgery can cause its own problems, as Josephine soon found out. Josephine and her son, Thomas, a Catholic priest, went to the surgeon recommended by Josephine's health-care plan. Father Tom remembers the meeting vividly to this day: "The surgeon presented a terribly dark picture: all doom and gloom. He said that in order to excise the tumor, he might have to cut several nerves, and she would never be able to swallow normally again, that she could not eat normal foods and her face would be permanently disfigured from the necessity to cut nerves controlling face muscles."

Both mother and son were stunned but unsure of the next step. On the bulletin board of a convent where he regularly said Mass, Father Tom put up a notice asking for prayers. Soon afterwards, a nun called him and reminded him that she was an audiologist, a technician who tests hearing. She said she worked for a top surgeon at New York University, Dr. Noel Cohen, who specialized in acoustic neuromas, but she wasn't sure if he would take their health insurance, HIP, which was from Josephine's husband's employment as a New York City bus driver. It turned out he did. Mrs. Petrillo met Dr. Cohen, and he painted a dramatically different picture. He would work with a renowned neurosurgeon, Dr. Joseph Ransohoff, to minimize any nerve damage. The one nerve that they absolutely had to cut governed muscles on the right side of the mouth. They tried an experimental technique to "glue" the severed nerve together, and when that didn't work (which took six months of healing to determine), they still didn't settle for second best, and they sent the patient to a third surgeon at NYU who specialized in nerve grafts. He harvested a nerve from the leg and put it under the tongue and into her face. Today, at age eighty-three, Josephine has almost completely normal nerves in her face, except for a slight asymmetry in her smile, particularly when she is tired. But otherwise she is fine.

HIP gave Josephine and her son a hard time, questioning how they had found out about the NYU doctor and refusing to cover the bill for the work by his teammate, the neurosurgeon. Father Tom wouldn't take no for an answer and made a series of calls to the insurer, finally landing at the desk of a vice president who told him, "We'll cover it. It was all a big misunderstanding." Father Tom said thanks, but had a pointed question, "What happens to the other little old ladies who don't have a priest son to advocate for them?" The vice president sighed, "Well, it is a problem."

Dealing with Insurance Companies

If your insurance company hassles you, my advice is this:

1. Obtain a copy of the insurance contract. Read it. Most state insurance commissioners now require plain English for these documents. Find out what your rights are under the contract and exercise them.
2. Don't take no for an answer. Many insurance companies seem to have coverage denials written into their business plan. They figure that most of their insureds will lack the gumption to challenge the first no. And they're right. This, of course, encourages even more aggressive denials of coverage by the insurance bean counters. You have to realize that placing obstacles in your path is just part of their profit plan.
3. Once you find out why the company won't pay, gather evidence to turn them around—your medical records and letters from the key doctors are important. Write the company an appeal letter with your evidence attached.
4. Write your state insurance commissioner a complaint if you exhaust your options with the company. Some commissioners

are in the industry's pocket, but some are genuine consumer advocates and can help you.

5. As a last resort, if your insurance coverage is connected to your job, you can file suit against the insurance plan in federal court under the ERISA law. If you win, the insurance plan has to pay your attorney fees. Some lawyers will accept these cases on a contingency fee, promising to charge you nothing for their time unless they win. If you need to take this step, make sure the attorney has experience in these kinds of lawsuits, which can be quite technical. It's guaranteed that your adversary at the insurance plan will have an experienced counsel.
6. The National Association of Insurance Commissioners has more useful information at http://www.naic.org/documents/consumer_alert_claim_denials.htm.[6]

Does Your Doctor Have a Conflict of Interest?

Most of the time we seek second opinions because we want more training, more expertise, and a fresh perspective brought to bear on our medical issue. One more special situation that calls for proceeding with caution and getting second or third opinions is when your doctor has a conflict of interest. Sometimes these conflicts are financial; it might turn out the doctor owns the machine he wants to run your body through. Sometimes the conflicts are more ego-driven—the doctor is bent on amassing the greatest number of cases using a technique he is pioneering, or he just wants to catch up with some colleagues in the volume of procedures of a particular type. Sometimes there are multiple sources of conflict. Ethical doctors are always supposed to put their patients' interests ahead of their own. But medicine is big business, and ethics sometimes take a back seat to the lure of money and prestige.

The main place where these conflicts exist today is with high-tech imaging machines where the doctors own the machine and "self-refer" patients for testing. Does the doctor want to test you for your own good? Or because he wants to meet the monthly payments on a million-dollar scanner? This is an acute issue now with a new technology called CT angiography, which uses high-speed CT scanners to take detailed pictures of the arteries that feed the heart. CT scanners have been around for decades, but only recently have they become refined enough to freeze a crisp image from the constant motion of a beating heart. Cardiologists can dazzle patients with the beauty of the pictures the scanners produce. Often, though, the CT angiography becomes just one more test, not a replacement, for the more traditional way that the heart is photographed, with dye squirted into the arteries through a catheter snaked up into the heart and then photographed in rapid movie-camera style with regular X-rays. That test has the disadvantage of requiring placement of these catheter tubes up into the heart, but it still produces the best pictures. So cardiologists and heart surgeons both rely on the catheter-based test to decide if you need treatment of the arteries with a balloon, a stent, or bypass surgery.

A turf war has been waging for the last decade, and shows no signs of truce, between radiologists and cardiologists about who should own these expensive CT angiogram machines.[7] Call me old-fashioned, but I think the best decisions are made when doctors are free of any financial interest. So cardiologists should use their best medical judgment in deciding what tests to recommend, but should not have any financial interest in the machines on which those tests are run.

I also think we patients should be pragmatic about this. When we go to the orthopedist and have an X-ray of the hip on a machine in his office, that's technically a conflict too, but a minimal one, as are simple blood-count tests and urine studies done in the back of the internist's office. (The maintenance and calibration of those machines in doctors' offices is another story, however; large laboratories usually do better because they have trained personnel who keep up the equipment.) Generally, my attitude is, nobody has to be as pure as the driven snow, but patients need to watch out for major conflicts, because doctors who have convinced themselves it is okay to "self-refer" will have a thousand rationalizations for some pretty dubious conduct.

A related conflict of interest is rampant at some of the most prestigious medical institutions; the lucrative consulting contracts that many medical professors have with drug and medical device manufacturers. (See Chapter 7, endnote 1 for more on this.) As long as they are disclosed to patients, these ties are not necessarily bad, but the medical industry is only beginning to make disclosure routine. The Cleveland Clinic made news at the end of 2008 by becoming the first institution to disclose on a Web site all its doctors' ties to industry, so patients can judge for themselves the objectivity of the advice that they receive.[8]

Discussing these conflicts directly with your doctor is unlikely to be productive. Virtually every physician I have met who receives any kind of freebies, be it a nice spread of poached salmon for the office staff's lunchroom or a few hundred thousand dollars in consulting fees, is shocked and offended—Shocked! Offended!—at the notion that his or her medical judgment could be influenced by something so mundane as money. As we discussed in Chapter 7, the truth is that any gift—even something as paltry as a pen—creates invisible tugs of obligation that interfere with the doctor giving you his or her best medical advice. The titans of the medical industry would not shower billions of dollars in "gifts" and "fees" on doctors if they did not think the money was purchasing something of value. Smart patients don't necessarily have to seek out only those doctors who are virginal of industry influence. After all, some doctors are sought out because they really are leaders in their fields, but we all need to know where the potential conflicts lie and take them into account when making our medical choices.

Getting Doctors Cooperating Instead of Competing Makes for Better Patient Care

Another "turf war" issue that patients need to be sensitive to can come up any time that your condition could be treated by different technologies, each in the domain of different specialties. Only a cardiac surgeon can put new blood-vessel-graft bypasses into your heart to repair the coronary arteries, and only a cardiologist can put in a stent to prop open your existing arteries. Which should you have? If a specialist tells you that you are better off with the other guy's technique, you can be confident of a disinterested opinion; if he tells you to sign up for his own type of surgery, you might want to at least see what the other guy says before making up your mind.

Cancer patients can hear such head-spinning conflicts of opinion—Radiation? Surgery? Chemo? Combinations thereof?—that advanced hospitals have committees called tumor boards, which bring all the relevant specialists to sit down together to try to develop a consensus about the best treatment for each individual patient. These tumor boards also bring together the most cutting-edge knowledge about cancer treatments, so if you have a newly diagnosed cancer, it's a good idea to find out if your case can be presented to one of these boards, to be reassured, if nothing else, that you are on the right course of treatment.

Outside of cancer, radiologists have expanded their expertise far beyond looking at pictures and telling some other specialist what appears to be wrong. The rapidly expanding field of interventional radiology involves repairing blood vessels from the inside by running tubes to the area needing treatment and doing surgery under continuous X-ray guidance. Sometimes that works out great and gives the patient a solid repair with much less cutting than traditional surgery. But other times disaster can strike when an interventional radiologist becomes too ambitious and tries to do things for which a surgeon should be called in.

Lyn Gross's Story: When Ambition Outruns Prudence

That happened to my client Lyn Gross. At age fifty-seven, she underwent a complex treatment by an interventional radiologist to repair a swollen artery, an aneurysm, at the base of her brain so that it wouldn't burst open and kill her. But the cure ended up worse than the disease: She suffered massive brain damage that left her confined to a wheelchair and in need of round-the-clock nursing care. What went wrong? The radiologist was originally supposed to limit his work to taking some detailed pictures of the swollen artery so they could be studied by a neurosurgeon and a radiologist; they could together decide if she would be better off with the surgeon's technique (drilling a hole in the skull and putting a clamp, or clip, on the swollen part of the artery from the outside of the vessel) or the radiologist's technique (sealing off the abnormal section of the artery from the inside of the vessel with tiny scaffolding—stents—plus nests of coiled-up wire). Both techniques were intended to block off the abnormal part of the artery while keeping the blood flowing through it to feed the brain. The radiologist instead talked the family into letting him go ahead with his type of treatment without any consultation with a neurosurgeon. Another wrinkle: The stent that he planned to use to hold open her artery had only been on the market for six months, so the track record was too short to have good evidence on who did well and who did poorly with the stent.

During the surgery, the radiologist ran into trouble because the stent didn't work. He had to seal off the entire artery that he had hoped to keep open. He assumed the loss of blood flow through this artery wouldn't harm her brain, but he didn't wake up the patient to make sure her brain was tolerating the alteration of blood flow he had caused. In the hours after he had finished his work and had moved onto another patient, Lyn Gross lay in an intensive care unit slowly suffering strokes on both sides of her brain, which the ICU staff didn't recognize because they did not realize that the artery the radiologist had blocked off was vital for feeding both sides of the brain. Had they known, she could have had treatment to boost the blood flow to the brain and reduce at least some of the damage from the blocked artery. The radiologist was busy with other patients while Mrs. Gross's brain damage gradually became irreversible.

No Team Plus No Plan Equals Patient Disaster

Lyn Gross's family didn't discover until it was too late that by the time of her procedure, a team approach for aneurysm treatment had developed at most major hospitals across the country, but not at the one where she was treated. Leaders in aneurysm treatment recognized that instead of having neurosurgeons and radiologists compete for business, patient by patient, the best way to sort through the specialist rivalries and give patients the most objective advice was to do two things: have patients meet with both kinds of specialists in the planning stage, and free up team members from having their income tied to how many cases they handle. Plus, it was recognized that since radiologists were not trained to provide postsurgery care, patients needed a team of neurosurgeons, neurologists, and specially trained nurses to deliver the right kind of care in the critical hours after a brain-artery intervention.

No effective team was there for Lyn Gross's aneurysm surgery, because the system had not been thought through by staff at the hospital where the radiologist operated on her. Instead, aneurysm patients were randomly assigned to one of five intensive-care units presided over by a single ICU "attending" who raced among the five units overseeing care given by residents in training for all different types of patients. Neither the attending nor the residents specialized in neurology or neurosurgery. The radiologist, when he finished with Mrs. Gross or his other patients, would jot a short note describing what he had done and then turn the patient over to an anesthesiologist to deliver the still-unconscious patient to the ICU. It was a system made for miscommunications and what in the jargon of medical error analysis is known as "handoff errors."

I found a good contrast at Johns Hopkins Hospital in Baltimore. When the neuroradiologist finishes a case, he wakes up the patient and makes sure the patient is neurologically intact. Then he walks the patient's gurney to the ICU and tells the staff exactly what happened. They jointly develop a plan for the post-op care. The ICU is limited to patients with brain issues, and doctors who staff it are "neurointensivists," a specialty that cross-pollinates neurology with intensive care. They are focused on the brain and look for treatable brain complications. Hopkins also has a team approach at the decision-making stage. They have neurosurgeons on staff who specialize in blood-vessel surgery in the brain ("cerebrovascular" surgeons), as well as interventional radiologists. Both neurosurgeons and radiologists talk to each other and the patient to decide which approach is the safest with the best chance of a good outcome. At the hospital where Lyn Gross was treated, by contrast, the radiologist had a busy practice treating hundreds of patients with wires inside the blood vessel, but the neurosurgeons on staff were all generalists who treated only the occasional aneurysm a few times a year. The imbalance in the volume of work meant that any patient referred to the hospital was likely to be steered toward the radiologist's practice rather than receive an objective evaluation. They say that to a hammer, everything looks like a nail. And the tool chest at this hospital for treating aneurysms only contained hammers.

Hopkins has a historic advantage. The first ICU of any kind in the United States was started there in 1923, as a three-bed unit for critically ill neurosurgery patients, by pioneering neurosurgeon Walter Dandy (the same surgeon who in 1937 first "clipped" an aneurysm). Hopkins had time and the resources to think through the ideal system for caring for patients who have just had brain surgery. At the hospital where Lyn Gross was treated, the system was cobbled together by hospital administrators who were trying to accommodate a revenue-generating feeder like the radiologist who operated on Mrs. Gross, without a lot of thought to what patients really needed.

Questions to Expose Conflicts of Interest and Lack of Teamwork

The painful lessons from Lyn Gross's case consist of a list of questions she and her husband had been too trusting to ask up front:

- Is there another kind of treatment with another doctor that might work for me? Can we set up a meeting with both doctors to sort out the pros and cons? (If you encounter resistance, even subtly, this should raise a question in your mind: Is this doctor giving me objective advice, or is he trying to steer me to the procedure that makes money for himself or his practice group and builds his roster of cases?)
- How well established are the different techniques that could treat me? (A complication rate that has been established over multiple years and thousands of patients is more reliable than a seemingly low complication rate for a new technique that might have collected data on only a few dozen patients.)
- If the doctor wants to use something new on me, how can I be assured it will be safer than a more tested technique?
- Has my doctor published his results in a peer-reviewed journal? How do they compare with others?
- How is the follow-up care organized? Where will I go after the operation, and what kinds of doctors and nurses will treat me? Are they specialists in my kind of condition?
- If something goes wrong, who will take care of me? Will it be someone who really knows about me? Will it be a specialist?

The really critical problem for Lyn Gross is that the radiologist did not allow the second opinion process to play out. He elbowed aside the neurosurgeon who sent Mrs. Gross to him for the brain artery pictures that were needed to decide the best course of therapy. Not knowing about turf wars between specialties and how teamwork is supposed to work, Mrs. Gross and her husband naively went along with a badly flawed plan in which the radiologist was planning to become, all by himself, the hero who cured her problem. His hubris proved fatal to her brain.

Something like Lyn Gross's story is played out every day in hospitals across the country, with all sorts of surgical procedures in all parts of the body. Patients are naturally attracted to what medicine calls "minimally invasive techniques"; when the window the surgeon cuts into the flesh is tiny, the scar is smaller and recovery is faster. So what's not to like? As we will see next in Chapter 10 with Jaime Vargas's story, when a surgeon uses a tiny camera and a video screen to see where he is supposed to be cutting, dreadful mistakes can be made, especially when the surgeon lacks solid experience with the minimally invasive technique.

Lifesavers:

Step Five Says Getting a Second Opinion Must Be Your First Choice

Whenever you stand at a major medical crossroads, you are best off consulting with multiple guides about which way you should travel. Sure, it's possible that the first person in a white coat who wanders by will know exactly how to guide you to where you need to go. But you will vastly improve your chances of finding the right treatment by seeing what different experts say. Once you know generally what the issue is, it is a good idea to hunt down a subspecialist. If it's a biopsy of your prostate, get a second look by a pathologist who looks at prostate all day long. If it's an MRI of your knee, have a musculoskeletal radiologist give another opinion. And if you are considering surgery, like Josephine Petrillo found out, you always want to find out if there are different techniques that reduce your chances of a bad result and maximize your chances of health. Once you pretty much know what you need, then it's time to move on to the next step in our Necessary Nine, finding the right surgeon.

10

When You Need Surgery: Avoiding Dr. Not-So-Good and Finding Dr. Right

When Jaime Vargas developed stabbing pains underneath his rib cage, he thought he might be having a heart attack. It turned out his gall bladder was inflamed because bile draining out of it had formed crystals and blocked the exit duct. Simple surgery was needed to take out the gall bladder. Twenty-two months later, after not one but two botched operations by the same surgeon, Jaime Vargas's liver was destroyed, and he died at age sixty-one. His widow and two grown children learned a painful lesson in the importance of avoiding a mediocre surgeon. Jaime Vargas's story introduces Step Six of our Necessary Nine steps, which is *"Choose a surgeon by experience and team structure, and learn the checklists for safe surgery."* In this chapter we will

> *Step Six:*
> **Choose a surgeon by experience and team structure, and learn the checklists for safe surgery.**

focus on choosing the right surgeon, and in Chapter 11, I'll tell you what else you need to know before you go under the knife, even once you have found Dr. Right and avoided Dr. Mediocre.

I'm not just mincing words when I say "mediocre" instead of "bad." Few doctors are so bad they should not be practicing. Jaime Vargas's surgeon was just mediocre. Mediocre doctors, like mediocre lawyers, are everywhere. Often, they cause no harm and actually help people. But the odds of being hurt badly or killed by a mediocre surgeon are much higher than with one practicing state-of-the-art medicine. How do you tell the difference? How do you avoid the dull and find the sharp? I offer some very personal guidelines developed from thirty years of experience with the whole spectrum of surgical quality. (Chapter 5, you will recall, focuses on finding the right doctor when you don't need surgery but need diagnosis and the correct medical management. The principles are similar, except listening skills are perhaps more important for a primary doctor who is the frontline diagnostician.)

When you're in an ambulance careening to the hospital, you have no time and no way to choose your doctor. If you have done advance research on the local hospitals (see Chapter 14), you might know enough to direct the ambulance where to take you. Even then, you will usually wind up with whatever doctor happens to be on call at that hospital at that time.

There are plenty of other occasions, though, when you do have the luxury of time to find Dr. Right. Yet most of us seldom make the effort, because we don't really appreciate the huge difference it can mean to end up under Dr. Wrong's knife, and we don't understand how many Dr. Wrongs are out there. Doing extensive research on potential doctors seems a little paranoid, a touch obsessive. So when I tell you a few stories about what can happen, I'm trying not to scare you, but to open your eyes to the work you need to do. And you will read about some patients who had happy endings thanks to the elbow grease they put into researching their surgeon ahead of time.

Jaime Vargas's Story

For his gall-bladder surgery, Jaime Vargas wound up with a surgeon in Cheverly, Maryland, a working-class suburb just east of Washington, D.C. This surgeon graduated from medical school in Istanbul, Turkey, in 1955 and finished his training in America in 1969. His profile at the Web site of the Maryland Board of Physicians, the state licensing and discipline agency, is unremarkable: no disciplinary actions, no court cases, no out-of-court settlements. (The case I brought against him isn't listed, because the Maryland licensing agency, in its wisdom, only mentions settlements if there have been three or more against the same doctor.) The clues that he was Dr. Wrong for Mr. Vargas were more subtle and easily missed.

The old-fashioned way to remove a gall bladder is by cutting a hole in the abdomen as wide as the palm of your hand; the surgeon can then directly see the gall bladder, a pear-size pouch nestled under the right side of the liver, and also can see its connection to the bile duct system. Bile, which is made in the liver and stored in the gall bladder, is essential to life, so preserving the bile duct that delivers it to the intestines is vital. When the gall bladder gets clogged up with crystallized bile, it can be surgically removed as long as the surgeon doesn't confuse the main highway from the liver to the intestines (the common bile duct) with the side road (the cystic duct) that connects the gall bladder to the common bile duct.

In the 1980s, surgeons developed a "minimally invasive" technique for a number of abdominal surgeries, cutting holes no wider than your thumb and inserting telescopes, called laparoscopes, into the belly so that the operative field appears on a video screen. Laparoscopic techniques can cut down on recovery time because far less trauma is done to the skin and musculature on the way in and out of the abdomen compared to the old "open" technique. But the downside is the surgeon cannot see as well what he is cutting, and there is a much higher risk of surgical error, particularly when a surgeon is new to the technique or has never been rigorously trained.

The surgeon who cut open Jaime Vargas certainly looked experienced. He had sprays of pewter at his temples, crow's feet at his eyes, and a late-middle-aged paunch—by his looks, not too old, not too young. But Jaime and his wife Monica didn't know that this surgeon had finished his training in general surgery many years before the technique that he used on Mr. Vargas was developed, and that his training for the technique consisted of a weekend session practicing on pigs followed by five operations on live patients with an instructor at his shoulder. And in fact, that's a fairly typical story for surgical innovation. New devices are adopted all the time for operations on the heart, brain, bones, and other organs with only minimal training for the operators. The only way you can find out how experienced your doctor is with a device he proposes to use on you is to ask. Most people, seduced by the idea of a smaller scar and a shorter hospital stay, don't ask.

After his training in the early 1990s in the minimally invasive technique, the surgeon hired by the Vargases used the laparoscope occasionally over the next several years before his encounter with Mr. Vargas in May 2000. But he never specialized in laparoscopic techniques or in surgery on the liver and gall bladder. He never joined any of the societies of surgeons specializing in laparoscopic surgery. As a general surgeon, he performed all kinds of procedures in the abdomen.

This surgeon had operated once before on Mr. Vargas, to take out a small cancer in his colon on the right side, near the liver. When the surgeon stuck the laparoscope into Mr. Vargas's belly on May 3, 2000, he found a lot of scar tissue from that old surgery obscuring his view. His surgical field was further obscured when a small blood vessel tore open. The surgeon grabbed what he thought was the cystic duct and cut it off, then fired two staples with a staple gun to seal the stump. He was wrong. He put the staples into the common bile duct, the tube he was supposed to protect, the tube that delivers the life-essential bile from the liver to the small intestine. He closed up the patient without realizing his error. Two days later, after Mr. Vargas became sicker and sicker, and tests showed he no longer had any bile in his intestines, the surgeon took the patient back to surgery and found his mistake and tried to fix it. But he had no experience in repairing bile ducts.

I met Jaime Vargas three months later on a muggy Washington August afternoon. Short and trim, he still looked younger than his fifty-nine years, his jet black hair only lightly flecked with salt. But he was still too weak after the two surgeries to return to his job fixing diesel engines on city buses for the Washington, D.C.–area transit system. He had just recovered from an episode where his repaired bile duct had become blocked and infected. The lack of good bile flow out of the liver had turned his eyes yellow from jaundice. When I saw him, though, he looked healthy enough that I gave him my standard talk about how if he recovered completely, we would probably not recommend pursuing a lawsuit. I explained that lawsuits are only for patients who have had such a medical disaster that their whole life has been permanently changed. We hoped that this jaundice episode would be his last and that he would recover eventually, as most people do who have bile duct repairs.

I didn't know then that Jaime Vargas was a dead man walking, that he would suffer repeated infections and blockages of his bile duct, that he would fall into a coma seventeen months later, and that he would die less than two years after his two surgeries. When a surgeon at Shands HealthCare at the University of Florida finally reopened his abdomen, he found a tangle of scar tissue and a half-dead liver. The original repair of the bile duct had been so poor that eventually most of the liver was destroyed by repeated infections and blockage of bile flow.

Which was no surprise, really, because when I asked him later how many bile ducts he had repaired before he had tried to fix the damage he did to Jaime Vargas, the first surgeon told me: only one in forty years of surgical practice in the Washington suburbs. Yet barely a forty-five-minute drive up the interstate is a team of bile-duct-repair specialists at Johns Hopkins Hospital in Baltimore; this team has done such repairs hundreds of times. Their work is posted in articles on the Internet[1] in which they boast of a 90-plus percent success rate. For a patient with an injured bile duct to be transferred into experienced hands takes just one phone call. That phone call could have saved Jaime Vargas's life. It's too bad neither he nor his wife knew to ask the right questions.

Here's another story, about a young couple who faced a life-threatening crisis for their toddler. Put yourself in the shoes of parents who are told their seventeen-month-old son has a tumor in his brain that must come out immediately. What would you do? In this case, polite but persistent questioning of doctors led to a happy outcome.

Josh's Story

Despite regular reassurances from their pediatrician, David and Cathy worried about their third child, Josh (all names have been changed at the parents' request). Josh was born in March 2005 with blue eyes, a shock of dark hair with blond tips, and skin that already looked tan. Josh was "the world's most easygoing baby," as David described him. But Josh didn't sit up on his own until he was nearly one year old, didn't crawl until he was fourteen months, and at sixteen months was nowhere near walking. He was way behind his older brother and sister. David knew that my son Brendan had a severe case of autism and had been diagnosed late, and in our work together on behalf of injured patients, he had seen firsthand the medical train wrecks that can happen when patients go along with a "probably nothing" diagnosis. Finally David called the developmental pediatrics program at a leading hospital in Washington, D.C. Consultations followed in short order with three neurologists, a physical therapist, a speech therapist, and others, as they worked through the dark possibilities of autism, genetic disorders, and neuromuscular problems. Nothing was found, and it looked like the optimistic pediatrician would be vindicated. But because of one nagging and very unusual thing—Josh's dominant left-handedness emerged long before most children show such a preference—he underwent an MRI scan of the brain and spine. Josh's tiny seventeen-month-old body was dwarfed by the giant metal donut that slowly drew him in.

Cathy, a mentally tough intensive-care nurse with years of experience caring for critically sick patients, was completely undone by the call she received from the neurologist. Cathy called David at work; she could barely talk through her tears. "Josh's got a brain tumor. He has to see the neurosurgeon this afternoon."

The neurosurgeon was soft-spoken but self-assured; he had handsome Nordic features. He explained that Josh had a growth about the size of a golf ball in his choroid plexus (the layer of brain substance on the surface of the ventricles where blood gets filtered into cerebrospinal fluid, which bathes and cushions the brain and spinal cord). The growth hadn't yet caused any blockage of flow in the cerebrospinal fluid, which can cause a buildup of high pressure and brain damage, but the surgeon said the ventricles (the fluid-filled spaces inside the brain) were already a little enlarged, and that made the situation more urgent. He told David and Cathy that he wanted to operate the next morning. The surgeon also said there was a good chance Josh would need a permanent tube implanted to carry fluid off the brain, which would create its own lifelong risks of infection and blockage.

David asked a key question: How often have you done this kind of operation with this kind of tumor? The answer: It was a rare tumor, and therefore, not since his training. He was a general neurosurgeon, not a pediatric specialist. David asked another key question: Was there any urgent need to operate the next day? The surgeon softened a bit and said no, but he added that if it were his family member, he'd want to proceed as quickly as possible.

So David and Cathy took one step back. They told the surgeon they would have to think about it. That night, they jumped on the Internet and called all their friends with medical knowledge. They looked for surgeons who regularly operated on children's brains and who knew about this choroid plexus growth. One name kept cropping up: a neurosurgeon at Johns Hopkins. The Hopkins surgeon had impressive credentials. He had not only finished a standard neurosurgery residency (itself the longest in medicine at nine years) but had also spent two years in a fellowship specializing in pediatric neurosurgery. The next morning, David called the surgeon's secretary (the number was an easy find on the Hopkins Web site) and told her that they needed to see him right away because another neurosurgeon said their son needed an immediate operation. David and Cathy found themselves in the Hopkins surgeon's office that same afternoon. He had a Mediterranean complexion and a perpetual five o'clock shadow. He, too, had a confident manner. He immediately gave them contrary advice to what they had heard in Washington. He said they didn't need to worry about Josh having a permanent shunt tube implanted; in his considerable experience with this tumor, which included two patients he'd operated on from Africa just a month before, a shunt would not be needed. The real worry, he explained, was that this growth could turn out to be cancerous, which would likely spell an early death for Josh. But they would only learn that once the growth had been removed and sent to the pathology lab for microscopic study.

The Hopkins surgeon also said there was no rush; they should just have it done sometime in the next few weeks. David and Cathy were grateful for the reprieve from the pressure they had felt from the other surgeon. They signed on with the Hopkins surgeon, and Josh had his surgery the following week.

The attentiveness of the surgeon to communication struck David. E-mails were returned within an hour (even David's request that trainees play as little role as possible in the surgery, which the surgeon politely declined). During the surgery, a nurse was sent out to brief the parents every twenty minutes. It went well, and soon they learned that no cancer cells had been seen.

David and Cathy had to stay alert right up until the moment Josh was sent home from the hospital. As they were preparing to leave, the senior neurosurgery resident (a doctor about eight years out of medical school) handed them a prescription for a thirty-day treatment with Decadron, a powerful steroid intended to keep down brain swelling after the surgery. Anybody who has taken steroids for poison ivy or a bad bee sting knows that the dose has to be tapered down rather than abruptly stopped when the pills run out. David questioned the lack of any taper on the prescription. The resident took the slip away and came back a few minutes later with a corrected prescription.

Seven days later, Josh was splashing in his neighborhood swimming pool. Three weeks later, he took his first steps. Over the next few months, Josh caught up with his age group and now is a normal preschooler in all respects.

What are the lessons from Josh's story? Is it brave or merely foolish to say no to a confident brain surgeon who wants to operate the next day? I vote for brave. David and Cathy had two very good reasons to take a step back from the commitment that was politely pressed on them by the first neurosurgeon. First, this was not an emergency where a day's delay would worsen Josh's condition. The key is that they had known enough—and felt comfortable enough—to ask a very specific question, thanks to a doctor friend who prompted them with the information that they faced an emergency only if the outflow of cerebrospinal fluid was blocked. (But even without that extra knowledge, a good question for any parent in their situation would have been, *Is it really an emergency? If so, why?*)

Second, David and Cathy knew they would likely be able to find another surgeon who had more experience in this kind of tumor, or at least someone who specialized in operating on children. Experience doesn't guarantee a better outcome, but it often helps. Even if they had elected to stay with the first surgeon after doing some independent research, they would have been able to face the surgery with the confidence of knowing that they had done their "due diligence" checking.

Josh's story also shows how important it can be for parents, spouses, and patients to follow their instincts and press for an answer when doctors keep saying, "It's probably nothing." If Cathy and David had let themselves be lulled by their pediatrician's reassurances, Josh's condition might not have been discovered until the window of opportunity for a happy result had been closed. One day, Josh will be able to read this story and thank his parents for being alert, keeping their wits about them under tremendous pressure, asking a lot of questions, and never giving up.

Finding Dr. Right: The Essential Questions to Ask—and the Answers You Need to Hear

There are two essential steps to finding a top surgeon: First, scout out names and check their backgrounds. Second, set up a meeting and talk to the surgeon face-to-face.

The Scouting Mission

Gathering names of potential surgeons is easy—too easy, because you can inundate yourself with names and run in circles. In descending order of reliability, here's what I recommend:

1. ***Any friend or family member who is a health-care professional should be asked to give you a short list of names based on their knowledge of the local medical scene.*** If they are close enough, ask them to work the phones and find out from anesthesiologists and operating-room nurses (the nonsurgeon professionals who watch every operation and so acquire a good sense of a surgeon's skills) what the scoop is on any doctor who makes your short list. Make sure they know the exact kind of surgery proposed for you, because one surgeon could be excellent for something else but not for what you need. Other knowledgeable insiders worth checking include "hospitalists" and critical-care doctors, who often are called in to treat the surgeon's patients after a procedure, and pathologists, who see the pieces of organs and tissues that the surgeon cuts out of patients in the OR.

2. ***The doctor who diagnosed the problem will have a referral network of surgeons to whom he has sent other patients.*** (But as you

will see later in this chapter, with stories like Susan Scoble's and Elmer Wischmeier's, this is not guaranteed to propel you to the top of the pack; you may have to take matters into your own hands.) One thing you want to watch out for is whether ties of friendship might interfere with your doctor's recommendation. My favorite question: "If it were your______[fill in as appropriate: spouse/child/parent], who would you want to do this surgery?"

3. *Check the Internet.* Start with the Web sites of the boards that certify surgeons who do this kind of surgery (and often there is more than one board because of an overlap between different specialties that do the same work). Start with the umbrella organization that oversees the major boards: the American Board of Medical Specialties.[2] Remember the warning in Chapter 5 (page 61) about "boards" that are not on the official list and may or may not have rigorous requirements to be certified. Another way I like to search for surgeons is to check Medline, the search engine of the National Library of Medicine (http://www.pubmed.com) for research published about the kind of surgery I am investigating.

If you try multiple scouting approaches like I recommend, you should start to see the same names coming up again and again. That is a very reliable sign. Here are a few more things to look out for:

1. Try to find a doctor who is within a day's trip. You will need to see this surgeon for follow-up visits, which can be just as important to a good outcome as skill with a knife.
2. To find the tip-top of the field, look for a doctor who not only specializes in the surgery you need but also has a long list of articles and lectures about the same surgery for his colleagues.
3. Focus on the institution where the doctor works. Good outcomes are as much a product of the surgical team—and the postoperative team—as the individual surgeon. If you hear that Dr. X has a God complex or is "brilliant but difficult," it should be at least a yellow flag, because some of the worst

errors happen when team members working with the doctor are too terrorized to speak up when they see a problem. You want to develop a sense (and this is sometimes hard to figure out in advance) that the surgeon works with a team of surgical assistants, nurses, and other caregivers who are all experienced and comfortable working with one another, and who deal with each other out of respect and not fear. (See the next chapter for more.) If you actually witness a doctor being abusive with staff, that's a bad sign for that doctor's quality of care.

4. Watch out for fancy titles that are more marketing hype than reality. Any doctor can rename his office the "Institute for the Advancement of XYZ Surgery" (just to make up a name that is not far off from many I have seen). Big hospitals are not immune from this, either. I will give you some questions next that will help you sort out who walks the walk from who merely talks the talk.

The Job Interview for Your Surgeon

Now that you have a short list, you have to talk to the doctor face-to-face. She will want you to bring with you any relevant imaging studies; you should also find out if the doctor needs to see anything else, like lab reports, and bring those too.

At this meeting, the surgeon is evaluating you (does your problem fall within her specialty, and can she really help you), and you are evaluating her. It may be intimidating to interview medical professionals as if you're hiring them for a job. But that is what you're doing, and it's often for the most important job of all: keeping you or a family member alive and healthy. Your main focus is on finding a surgeon who has operated on many people just like you, and so knows all the techniques that separate a so-so result from an excellent one, and who also has built a team that is relentlessly focused on all the tiny details that need to be executed—before, during, and after the surgery—to produce the healthiest outcome.

So here is a list of questions to ask—and answers you need to hear—from any surgeon who may be performing a procedure on you:

1. "Do I really need any surgery?" (A busy surgeon—and busy means a lot of doctors have confidence in this surgeon—will be more candid than a surgeon with time on his hands to tell you that waiting might be the most prudent thing to do. For everything except purely cosmetic surgery, the general rule is if you don't really, really, really need surgery, you don't need surgery.)
2. "What is the exact procedure that you would recommend for a family member if they had the same thing I have?" (You need to make sure the surgeon and you are both talking about the exact kind of procedure proposed for you, not some close cousin.)
3. "Who would you ask to do the operation on a close family member of yours if you couldn't?"
4. "How often do you do this kind of procedure?" You want to hear "every week" (and if you hear "a few times a year" or less, you want to drop this surgeon).
5. "Is there anyone at your institution (in your partnership, in my town, etc.) who does these procedures more than you do? If so, would you mind if I speak to him or her?" (A defensive response to this question is a red flag.)
6. "How long have you been doing this procedure?" (Be careful with this one, because a surgeon like Mr. Vargas's gall bladder doctor could honestly answer "years" but have less experience in volume of cases than a fresh-faced young surgeon who has just finished rigorous subspecialty training at a major teaching hospital with several cases every week. The more important focus is volume of recent cases.)
7. "Do you have fellowship training in this procedure?" (This is not a deal breaker but it is good to know. A fellowship is what comes after residency when the surgeon wants deeper training in a subspecialty; it typically involves one or two years of intensive hands-on work at the side of a top surgeon.)

8. "What are the most common problems that happen with this surgery? What do you do to keep them to a minimum? How often do they happen even when everyone is careful?" (See Chapter 11.) (Anyone who says, "I've never had a complication," or "There is no risk," is not telling the truth and should be avoided.)
9. "What is your surgical wound infection rate? How does that compare to other surgeons at your hospital?" (This is a good marker for a meticulous surgeon; he or she should take pride in a very low rate. See Chapters 11 and 13.)
10. "Who is going to do the critical parts of my surgery?" (This is important whenever you are in an institution that trains new doctors. You have a right to decline to have these trainees practice on you. You also have a right to have a particular surgeon do the critical work. On the "informed consent" that you sign before surgery, look for any language like "I give consent to Dr. Right or his designee to do the following operation," and just cross out the part about "or his designee.")
11. "Who will be in charge of my postoperative care? If it's not you, the surgeon, why not? How often can I expect to see you while I'm still in the hospital?" (See the discussion of Lyn Gross's case in Chapter 9.)

People can feel awkward asking these important questions, especially if you were raised to show deference to anyone wearing a white coat. That's why it can be crucial to have an advocate present, sometimes just a family member who is knowledgeable about medicine, other times the official hospital "patient advocate." (You'll find out more about this in Chapter 12.) And there are polite ways to ask pointed questions. My favorite way to ask, as you'll notice on the list above, is like this: "If the operation were being done on your______ [fill in as appropriate: spouse/child/parent], who would you want to do it?" Another way to ask: "If we wanted to get a second opinion from someone with even more expertise than you have, who would you recommend?"

If the surgeon doesn't have time for these questions, that is not the surgeon for you. I don't care how long the resume is or how fancy the surgeon's reputation is.

Now, if a major complication happens in the first surgery, you have to go back to square one in deciding what happens next. When there has been a complication of surgery and a repair is needed, it's only natural to assume, as the Vargases did, that the first surgeon will be the one to clean up his own mess, so to speak. But there's no such rule. It is critically important to be assertive after a surgical complication. That starts with finding out exactly what happened. Mr. Vargas never got a clear idea from his surgeon. Another doctor finally told him. Mr. Vargas recalled the moment vividly for me because the explanation was so simple and cleared up months of confusion; his eyes widened as he said, "He told me that my surgeon cut the connection between the liver and the rest of my body! My goodness!" Had he known that this first mistake was so basic, and so huge, and had he learned that the same surgeon had next to no experience in repairing severed bile ducts, Mr. Vargas would have had the motive to find someone else to fix the error.

Searching for Dr. Right is something that knowledgeable patients do all the time. When a celebrity gets a serious disease, people hardly notice when the celebrity does some doctor shopping. In 2008, when he discovered he had brain cancer, Senator Ted Kennedy easily could have sought treatment at the hospital where the cancer was found—the Massachusetts General Hospital in Boston, one of the country's oldest and most prestigious medical institutions, staffed by faculty members of Harvard Medical School. But Kennedy cranked up his telephone network and eventually flew to North Carolina to undergo surgery with Dr. Allan Friedman, the chief neurosurgeon at Duke University Hospital. News accounts of his decision talked about Friedman's superb reputation for pioneering the aggressive and successful treatment of hard-to-reach tumors deep in the brain. The news stories also talked about the quick rapport that Senator Kennedy developed with Friedman when they first talked on the telephone. One piece of advice that Kennedy received from a top neuro-oncologist (brain-cancer specialist) at the National Cancer Institute, Howard Fine, could apply to anyone: "Talk to several surgeons, and find where you feel most comfortable."[3]

"Well," I can hear you saying, "that's all fine for a United States senator with a famous family name. Sure, the surgeons are going to fall all over themselves to return his calls. Fat chance of that happening for me and my family!" If you think that, you're wrong! Top surgeons are only an e-mail or phone call away. True, you may not reach the top banana immediately, but you can definitely reach the top assistant and schedule an appointment. To prove this, and to emphasize how important it is to assertively shop for a top surgeon, let's look at some success stories of regular people I know.

How a Librarian Found the Right Surgeon and Proved She Wasn't Ready to Die

When Susan Scoble moved to Houston in 2001, she knew she was starting a new life and a new job after a divorce. What she didn't know is that her move would save a life too—her own. The symptoms started around Christmas 2001 with a constant burning in her stomach. Antacids didn't help. She went to doctors who put a camera down her throat to peer around the stomach, but they found nothing. They told her it was probably acid reflux. After six months with worsening pain that had spread to between her shoulder blades, she told her internist that she felt she was dying, and he had to do something. He sent her for an ultrasound of her abdomen, where sound waves give a picture of internal organs. Around the same time, she noticed the whites of her eyes had yellowed. It was a few days before Memorial Day 2002.

Susan picks up the story:

"I knew by the technician's face doing the ultrasound that he had found something bad. I was told to go to my internist's office immediately. It seemed to take forever for him to come in to talk to me. I remember thinking, *He is taking his time to work up his courage to tell me something bad.* When he walked in, he immediately went over to an anatomy diagram on the wall and pointed to the pancreas. He said you have pancreatic cancer and again pointed to the diagram and tried to explain to me where it was located. I couldn't have cared less where it was. I was in shock. I remember asking, 'Is it bad?' His response to me was it is one of the deadliest cancers to have, with fewer than 5 percent living more than two to three months."

He said all this, she remembers, "with no emotion or concern." But he did send her to a surgeon because the yellowing in her eyes signaled jaundice, which meant that the tube delivering bile from her liver to her intestines had become blocked by the cancer pressing on it. Bile is necessary for life, and she wouldn't live even two to three months if the tube couldn't be reopened.

After the surgery, at Susan's bedside, the surgeon kept his eyes on the floor. He seemed in a hurry to leave. The surgeon gave her no more hope than the internist had. He had been able to put a metal tube into the bile duct to keep it open, but the cancer itself, he told her, was inoperable because it had wrapped around a major vein carrying blood from the liver. He, too, said she had no more than a few months to live. Susan felt herself standing at the bottom of a dark pit with no way out.

Just then, her two grown sons arrived with a ladder and a flashlight.

Bill and Brad Scoble would not accept the grim prognosis for their mother. They insisted on another opinion from the nearby M.D. Anderson Cancer Center, a world-class cancer research and treatment facility. Patients could go there on their own, but a doctor's referral could speed the way. So they called back Susan's internist. He told them they were wasting their time. Treatment at Anderson would be no better than his own small suburban hospital could offer. But if they demanded it, he would refer them.

Susan hit bottom as she awaited the appointment at Anderson. "There are no words to describe the feeling you have when you are told you are going to die. Nothing in life seemed to matter." She told herself that if she could find just one person who had survived pancreatic cancer, maybe she could muster some hope for the battle her sons urged on her. And then it happened: One day, a television show called *Houston Medical* featured a woman who had been told, just like Susan, that her pancreatic cancer was inoperable. But with the help of some doctors at Anderson, the tumor was shrunk to an operable size and then was removed, and she lived to tell about it.

A few days later, Susan felt like pinching herself when she found herself sitting across a desk from one of the doctors featured on the TV show. He was an oncologist who specialized in pancreatic cancer. The oncologist said, yes, the tumor was inoperable in its current state, and he could not make any promises, but they could try to shrink it to a manageable size with drugs and radiation. The oncologist gave her three treatment options. Susan took the most aggressive option. As she puts it, "I called him my general and told him we were going to fight the battle." She tolerated the treatment so well that she could continue working as a law-school librarian and even took online courses for her master's in library science. Then, in April 2003, after many rounds of chemo, radiation, and experimental-drug protocols, the tumor was small enough to chance the surgery, although still very close to the portal vein.

Susan remembers meeting the surgeon to plan the operation. "All I could do was stare at his hands. I thought to myself, *He will hold my life in these hands.* He had a very gentle, kind air about him. After my surgery was successful, I told him, 'Thank you for saving my life,' and he said he did not do anything, he was just the carpenter."

This was not the end of Susan's story. The surgeon warned her that the pancreatic cancer could return, and with a vengeance, because it could transform itself to render the chemotherapy drugs used on the first round impotent for the next round. So she submitted to a CT scan every three months, her body slowly sliding into the donut-shaped machine as X-rays danced around her belly, looking for new shadows. Three years later, the radiologist spotted a suspicious shadow in one lung. It turned out to be a cancer nodule, but it, too, was removed successfully by another Anderson surgeon, a lung specialist, in December 2007.

Today, years after she was told she had three months to live, Susan Scoble rolls on the floor with three gifts that her sons presented her after the cancer diagnosis: grandchildren William, Abbie, and Alyssa.

Pancreatic Cancer Resources

Susan Scoble recommends three resources for patients with pancreatic cancer:

1. PANCAN (http://www.pancan.org) Pancreatic Cancer Action Network. Says Susan, "They provide information about pancreatic cancer, hospitals, doctors, and success stories."
2. A pancreatic discussion board provided by Johns Hopkins (http://www.pathology.jhu.edu/pancreas_chat/).
3. A podcast called Patient Power with Andrew Schorr (http://www.mdanderson.org, click on Patient Power). "This talk show represents the patient's point of view and connects to M.D. Anderson medical experts, inspiring patients, survivors, and family members."

She gives credit widely: to her sons for prodding her into seeking out the doctors at Anderson; to her friends and family and coworkers for supporting her through hard times, especially her friend Barbara, who drove four hours each way every other Friday for ten months to sit with Susan through chemo sessions; even to her ex-husband, for helping out through some of the lowest spots. She credits her pastor, in those early dark days, for telling her, "You can try to hide from it and feel sorry for yourself, or you can face the enemy and give it your best fight." Susan also credits prayer groups at many churches for keeping her on their prayer lists. And as you might expect, Susan is filled with praise for M.D. Anderson. She says, "I found that having cancer can be a curse, but it can also be a blessing. I cannot tell you how many good things have happened to me since I was first diagnosed. I found M.D. Anderson to be a place filled with people fighting to live, not a place that I feared at first of dying people. These men, women, and children go to battle every day to fight this enemy called cancer. Their stories are full of hope because most of them do not want to give up. I have met such wonderful people at Anderson."

But she adds this: "I did learn that I had to be my own patient-advocate. I learned which areas at Anderson were the nicest for scans and gave the best service, I learned that lab work can be done a few days prior to appointments at slow times with no wait, I learned to always check when chemo is given to make sure it is the right kind, and I learned to always question when lab procedures were requested, what kind and why. Mostly I learned not to be afraid to ask questions or to speak up; after all, it was my life."

A Farmer Gets World-Class Care: Elmer Wischmeier's Story

Still not convinced that you as a regular person can win world-class medical care? Then consider one more story. This one starts at the front gate of a family farm in the Midwest—not the neighborhood where you would first look for sophisticated treatment. But when you are a patient seeking out the best care, where you live is less important than how much you want to live.

Point your car north from Louisville, Kentucky, and you will quickly cross the Ohio River into the limestone hills of south-central Indiana, and about an hour from Louisville you will come to the town of Seymour, Indiana, population 19,000. Hang a left on U.S. 50 and soon you will find the farm of Elmer and Dolores Wischmeier. Elmer Wischmeier has tilled the land for nine decades. He is from a family of German immigrants; his father, too, farmed the land. Elmer grew corn, soybeans, and wheat—and raised cattle, hogs, chickens, and a few sheep—until finally at age eighty-eight, he rented out the last ten acres he had been farming and decided to content himself with a big vegetable garden.

The year he finally climbed off the tractor, Elmer grew sick over the summer. He lost his energy and began to complain of stomach pains. This was a man who had not been sick a day in his life. An MRI was performed in September 2004 at the only hospital in the county, and that revealed a golf-ball-size tumor in his liver.

No one can live without a liver. The liver produces the proteins that make blood clot; it processes drugs and has a thousand other vital functions. But here is one secret that surgeons know, which many nonsurgeon doctors don't appreciate: The liver is the one organ in the body that can regenerate itself. A surgeon can cut out as much as three-fourths of the liver, and the remaining part, if it's healthy, will regrow to a full liver.

Not knowing this, and not knowing the success that surgeons have developed over the last decade in curing liver cancer by cutting out wedges of the liver, Elmer Wischmeier's local internist was ready to give up. He thought that chemotherapy was the only option but said it would be too hard on Mr. Wischmeier at age eighty-eight. He did offer a second opinion, and sent the family to a medical oncologist in the nearby city of Columbus, Indiana. The oncologist said the same thing: It was time to give up.

Priscilla Wischmeier, at age forty-nine the youngest of the Wischmeier's four children, works as a paralegal for an attorney in Seymour, Indiana, who represents victims of defective products. When her father received the gloomy news, Priscilla knew nothing about the liver, nothing about cancer, and little about medicine. But she has an inquisitive mind and a fighting spirit, and her legal work made her comfortable with reaching out to experts across the country.

Priscilla still vividly remembers her high school days working with her father on the farm: disking the ground, baling straw, cultivating the fields. She knew, as the closest grown daughter, that it was time for her to step up again and help.

"I wasn't ready to accept what the local doctors told me; I needed to hear it from someone with expertise and to know that I had done everything I could," she says. "The Sunday after Thanksgiving 2004, I began to search for liver-tumor specialists. The first Web site that came up was http://aboutlivertumors.com. I skipped over it at first, thinking that it would be in Texas or Philadelphia or some faraway place. After searching for several hours, I finally went back to that first Web site to find out where they were located. Much to my surprise, these physicians are at the University of Louisville. Dr. Kelly McMasters is a professor of surgical oncology at the University of Louisville. The Web site at that time provided an e-mail address directly to him, so I thought, *Why not?* I e-mailed him about my dad, and within two hours he responded that he was in Phoenix for a medical conference but that if I called their office on Monday morning, his associate, Dr. Charles Scoggins, would see my dad on Thursday. It was like a miracle! Dr. Scoggins said it was in fact a malignant tumor and the best course of treatment was removal. After extensive pre-op evaluation my father had surgery the second week of December. Most of the right lobe of his liver was removed. He lost no blood, was only in the hospital five days and while the recovery process was lengthy for a man of eighty-nine years, he is still alive and healthy today."

The Wischmeiers were amazed at the attentiveness of Dr. Scoggins. He was professional, patient, and kind, and he wanted to make sure he answered every one of the family's questions. After the first meeting, Elmer's wife, Dolores, commented, "Now, that's a real doctor." After Dr. Scoggins took out the cancer, he came to the hospital room at least once and sometimes twice a day. He gave the family his pager number. They found from repeated experience that all phone calls were returned in ten minutes. Because Dr. Scoggins was from Texas, Elmer liked to tease him; he wanted to know how many oil wells Dr. Scoggins owned. (For the record, none.)

Elmer Wischmeier, age ninety-three at this writing, remains a big, sturdy man, with one of those sly smiles that let you know he is in on the joke. He plays his favorite card game of euchre almost every day, drives his car, and maintains a huge garden with sweet corn, green beans, tomatoes, onions, cabbage, green peppers, broccoli, sweet potatoes, and turnips. He plants a few pumpkins every fall. He enjoys taking the great-grandchildren out to the barn and watching them frolic in the hayloft. He and Dolores celebrated their sixty-first wedding anniversary, then Dolores took sick and died as this book was going to press. Elmer has a hole in his heart from losing her but remains active still.

Priscilla's conclusion could be the coda for this book: "Resources are only as limited as we let them be." Amen to that.

Before we leave the Wischmeier story and Susan Scoble's before it, I want to add one caveat: Do not conclude that going to a large medical-school-affiliated hospital is necessarily the way to find the best care for your condition. Chapter 14 is essential reading about how to compare hospitals and how to know when you need the brand-name institution or might be better off with the local option.

Surgical Procedures with the Highest Rates of Preventable Injuries

(This is a useful list from a well-regarded medical-quality researcher, Atul Gawande of Harvard. The items are ranked in descending order, with the percentage of preventable adverse events.)[4]

Leg blood-vessel bypass graft	11.0 percent
Abdominal aortic aneurysm repair	8.1 percent
Colon resection	5.9 percent
Open-heart surgery (bypass and valve replacement)	4.7 percent
Transurethral resection of bladder or prostate cancer	3.9 percent
Gall-bladder removal	3.0 percent
Uterus removal	2.8 percent
Knee/hip replacement	2.6 percent

Lifesavers:

Step Six—Tracking Down a Top Surgeon

Once it's clear you need surgery, Step Six of our Necessary Nine steps bears down on how to find Dr. Right and steer clear of Dr. Mediocre (and then, in the next chapter, the further essential ingredients for safe surgery). Your task is simple but takes some work; you want to find, reasonably close by, the surgeon with the most experience treating exactly the condition you have. This surgeon also should have assembled a close-knit team that helps maximize the positive outcomes. Your mission has two parts: first, the scouting expedition where you gather names of prospective surgeons; and second, the job interview where you make the final decision. A good scout shakes a lot of trees—friends and family, especially if they have a medical background, and most especially if they work in or near operating rooms so have firsthand knowledge of who wields the knife with the most skill; your primary-care doctor (but watch for whether bonds of friendship influence her recommendations); and the Internet, which will open a window onto who does cutting-edge research about the kind of condition you have. You should start seeing the same names over and over, and then you can decide whom to go talk to. Look at the final caveats, pages 129–130, before you make your final interview picks. The interview itself takes gumption; you will be face to face with a white-coated, gray-templed eminence, but remember, your questions are vital because you are hiring someone for the most important job of all, saving your life. So, using my list of eleven key interview topics, pages 131–132, write out your questions in advance, take an ally with you, and make sure you ask enough to satisfy yourself that this is Dr. Right. If the surgeon plays the intimidation card and brushes off your questions, you should cross the surgeon off your list, no matter how imposing his paper credentials are. The real Dr. Right will give you plenty of time to explore all your questions, calm your fears, and build your trust in the intimate relationship you are about to begin.

11

Making a List and Checking It Twice: The Key to Safe Surgery

Before any airplane in America takes off, the pilot and copilot go through long checklists that cover every system. The mechanics have already been through their safety checklists. Only when everything is checked off can the plane lumber onto the runway. After all, the safety of every flight depends on a complex interplay between human and machine.

Early in the twenty-first century, some sixty years after the airline industry figured this out, safety checklists have now arrived in the operating room. Too many bodies have piled up in the meantime. And too many ORs still practice in an unquestioning "the surgeon is God" way, which has led to so many preventable injuries. The good news is that patients can use their own checklists to help their chances of staying safe with surgery. This applies even if you have followed the advice in the last chapter and have found a top surgeon with whom you are comfortable, because most of the problems we will focus on in this chapter are not failures of individual technique but team errors, or in the current jargon, "systems failures." When the patient becomes an active part of the team, that helps cut down on these systems failures. That's why the second part of Step Six of our Necessary Nine focuses on making you a part of the team so that you can help make sure that what is known to work for safe surgery happens with your case.

Just about anything can go wrong in an operating room. Some mishaps can be marked down to fate, but many allow no excuse. One patient gets an operation intended for another patient. The surgeon removes the patient's only healthy kidney instead of the cancerous kidney that needed to come out (this happened at Methodist Hospital in suburban Minneapolis in 2008,[1] to a child in Ireland in 2008,[2] to an elderly woman in Nashville in 2006,[3] and to a young man in Wales in 2000[4]). The patient is set on fire by an electrical device used to seal off blood vessels. An organization called the National Quality Forum has put together a list of twenty-eight "never events"—events that should never happen but do happen distressingly often. I'm reprinting the list in an appendix (see page 261) because it's useful information for us patients. To know that something should never happen helps arm us both before and after: before, to watch for what the hospital does to make sure things don't happen; and after, if they don't, to raise hell.

These wrong-kidney surgeries, to take one example, all would have been prevented if the X-ray images showing which was the healthy kidney and which was the diseased one had been brought to the operating room with the patient. Of course, it's not the patient's fault that the X-rays weren't in the operating room. Forewarned, however, is forearmed, and now you know that if you are undergoing any surgery that depends on X-rays to localize the correct site, it is a good idea to ask your surgeon to make sure to have the X-rays handy to double-check before the first cut.

Is it too much to ask patients to know these things and remind their surgeons? Of course it is. If medicine had a long-standing culture of safety like the aviation industry, it would be entirely unnecessary for patients to be so vigilant. But medicine has a long way to catch up, and in the meantime patients can help to protect themselves. Patients, after all, have one advantage over airline passengers; the safety checks on patients are all done in our presence, and until the moment we are knocked out by anesthesia, we can watch and see everything that is happening.

"Sign the Site" and Prevent Mix-ups Like Karen's

My client Karen Bellas would have avoided receiving the wrong surgery on her left foot if the X-rays had been in the operating room. The surgeon, a prominent foot surgeon at Georgetown University Hospital in Washington, D.C., operated on the correct foot. That much was obvious from the bump on top of her foot that was painfully chafing her shoe and needed to be cut out. But the surgeon also gave her an extra procedure that she didn't need. He realigned her big toe by breaking it and fusing it to the forefoot with a screw, a procedure that patients only need when the big toe splays in the wrong direction when walking. An X-ray of the patient standing up shows the problem clearly, but when the patient is lying on a gurney, it's not that obvious. So Karen was ripe for being confused with another patient, especially since the surgeon followed his usual practice of lining up several patients for back-to-back procedures to fill his allotted window of OR time. Karen, a nurse who then tended to homeless men at a free clinic in the Adams-Morgan neighborhood of D.C., was left with a painful deformity that required an extra surgery and still left her unable to walk distances without pain.

Karen's permanent injury (a combination wrong-site, wrong-patient mishap) also could have been averted if her surgeon had followed a guideline first put out in 1997 by the American Academy of Orthopaedic Surgeons. The surgery group recommended that surgeons follow this drill with each patient:[5]

1. Review with the patient and the operating-room personnel what procedure is planned. This should happen before the patient receives any sedative drugs, so the patient can be alert enough to participate.
2. Write the surgeon's initials with indelible ink on the patient's body at the operative site.
3. Review the patient's chart in the operating room before starting the surgery.

Helen's Story

Wrong-site surgery is only one of the things that can go dreadfully wrong on the operating table. My client Helen F. (her last name has been omitted at her family's request) is proof that something can happen even worse than death. In October 2004, at age thirty-four, Helen, a real-estate agent who had emigrated from Lebanon, underwent cosmetic surgery at a spanking new outpatient surgery center in Rockville, Maryland. She wanted to trim her Middle Eastern nose and also lose some fat from her neck. Her heart stopped for twelve minutes on the table, and the thinking parts of her brain suffocated from lack of oxygen. Today, years later, she lives in a bed in her mother's living room on a quiet cul-de-sac. She looks but does not see, flails her arms but cannot communicate, eats and drinks only through surgical tubes. Helen is caught somewhere between what doctors call a "persistent vegetative state" and "minimal consciousness," a limbo between life and death.

I went to the surgery center a year after the episode to find out what happened. It wasn't clear from the medical records. (And unlike the aviation industry, there is no independent agency for health-care facilities that investigates and files a public report of what went wrong when a catastrophe has happened.) One by one, I took depositions from the surgeon, an impatient, arrogant man who had convinced himself that something in Helen's body had just reacted in a bizarre way to the standard drugs he used to numb the flesh; the nurse who acted as the "circulator," preparing all the drugs that went into the patient; and the nurse anesthetist who gave general anesthesia. Each of them, it turned out, had a completely different idea of the amounts and concentration of the local anesthetic drugs injected by the surgeon into her neck and nose.

The anesthetist was supposed to act as the safety officer to protect her unconscious patient. The anesthetist, however, assumed without inquiring that the surgeon was using a highly diluted solution for the local anesthetic. The dilute solution is standard for suctioning fat from under the skin. But the surgeon had asked the circulating nurse to prepare a full-strength mix of short-acting and long-acting local anesthetic drugs to help the surgery go faster and give the patient post-operative comfort. Twenty minutes after he injected the neck, her heart slowed and then stopped beating. An expert told me that the surgeon had simply anesthetized the heart with a whopping overdose of local anesthetic drugs; they traveled from the circulating blood to the heart and blocked the conduction of electrical signals into the muscle fibers, preventing the heart from beating. Once the anesthetic drugs eventually washed out, her heart recovered, but in the meantime her brain was asphyxiated.

One standard piece of the anesthesia-safety culture is to assume nothing in the operating room. When a surgeon orders a drug, the person who fills the order recites back what he heard. When the surgeon starts to administer the drug, the surgeon is supposed to announce exactly what he is giving, and if he doesn't, the anesthesiologist stops the surgeon and asks. It's a simple way to prevent tragic miscommunications. Helen's plastic surgeon, who owned the operating suite, decided not to bother with having an MD anesthesiologist on-site. That would have made his cosmetic surgery prices less competitive. He also chose not to hire an anesthesiologist as a consultant to develop standard safety protocols. Those protocols are required by Medicare for any surgery center that wants to be eligible for reimbursement. But this piece of paperwork was delegated to a junior surgeon, and at the time of Helen's case, no protocol was yet in place. In fact, the surgery center wasn't accredited either by Medicare or by any of the three private agencies that inspect and accredit freestanding surgery centers. Helen never thought to ask about accreditation. Working without accreditation, I found out, was perfectly legal in Maryland, as long as the facility didn't try to bill an insurance company. (There's a question for state lawmakers: How is it that insurance companies have more safety protection written into the laws for them than patients paying their own bills?)

Helen's case illustrates something that safety analysts in high-risk enterprises often see. It's never just one thing that goes wrong to cause a tragedy. A series of slips, errors, oversights, and misunderstandings occur together. In the trade, they call it cascade analysis. If only the medical director had instituted a policy about handling drugs in the OR. If only they had hired an anesthesiologist to set up their procedures. If only the surgeon had called out exactly what he wanted. If only the circulating nurse had done her job. If only the anesthetist had asked what was being injected into Helen's neck.

And you could add to that: If only Helen had asked if the facility was accredited. If only she had known enough to ask to have a medical-doctor anesthesiologist present for her anesthesia, not a nurse. She is in no way at fault for what happened. But once we understand that it takes half a dozen errors to cascade together to produce an injury, and that it only takes one correction in that process to set things right, we can see that patients can play a vital, necessary role in keeping their medical ship on a smooth and happy course.

For patients, asking if the surgery center is accredited needs to become as second nature as asking if the surgeon is board-certified. Thousands of surgery centers now operate in the United States. Patients like them for the convenience, and insurance companies like them because they usually cost less than hospitals. Are they cheaper because safety corners are being cut? That was true for the surgery center where Helen's life was ruined. For all the dangers of hospitals (see Chapters 12 and 14), every major hospital submits to regular accreditation reviews and has, among other features, a chief of surgery, a chief of anesthesiology, and a committee that reviews injury events, all of which make it a safer place. Surgery centers can be as safe as hospitals, but at the least, only when they follow the requirements of an accreditation agency.

Who Will Put You to Sleep in the OR? You Need to Ask

A further word about who puts you to sleep in the operating room: The practical realities of modern surgery don't allow every operating room to have an MD anesthesiologist running the care. Nurse anesthetists can do an excellent job. At a minimum, though, they need close oversight by an anesthesiologist who is running no more than a handful of ORs in the same building at any one time. Before the day of the surgery (it's too late if you wait until the same day), you need to ask these questions:

1. Who is giving anesthesia to me? What are their qualifications?
2. If it's a nurse, is she certified as a nurse anesthetist?
3. Will there be an MD anesthesiologist nearby on the premises if something goes wrong?

Do not let the facility talk you out of these minimum requirements by telling you, "We're not giving you full anesthesia. It will just be light sedation." (Another term is *conscious sedation.*) Any amount of sedation that is enough to make you comfortable enough to have tubes thrust into your body is also enough to compromise your airway, interfere with your breathing, or affect your heart.

My own preference is for the anesthesiologist to give me his full time and attention. They say that giving anesthesia consists of hours of boredom punctuated by moments of terror. Just in case terror happens, I want the most knowledgeable and best-trained person right there with me. If you agree, and if you inquire early enough, you can insist on the same level of protection.

A Safe-Surgery Checklist

The World Health Organization, part of the United Nations, has a safe-surgery project with a surgery checklist that I've adapted here. These are essential items that the health-care personnel must attend to before you are knocked out. This checklist applies to almost all surgeries. You might want to talk to your surgeon and the anesthesia provider about the items on this list. If the surgeon and the anesthesiologist are *not* planning on having *all* of these items done for your surgery, you deserve to know if there's a good reason. I'm focusing on the aspects of the checklist that will be visible to you when you go in for the surgery, but if you don't ask about them ahead of time, it may be too late to back out.

All of the following things need to happen *before* you undergo anesthesia:

1. Someone should confirm with you your identity, the type of procedure you're having, the site of the surgery on your body, and your consent to have it done. Do all these questions seem irritatingly obvious? The WHO says, "While it may seem repetitive, this step is essential for ensuring that the team does not operate on the wrong patient or site or perform the wrong procedure."[6]
2. The surgeon should mark the operative site with her initials using a permanent marker–type pen.
3. The anesthesia equipment needs to be inspected to make sure everything is working and they have enough supplies of emergency medications. (You are unlikely to notice this unless you ask the anesthesia provider.)
4. A pulse oximeter should be placed on one of your fingers and should be functioning. If you're normal, you'll score between 95 and 100 percent. With 100 percent "oxygen saturation," all of your red blood cells have oxygen molecules attached to them. (I'm still haunted by a case involving a broken pulse oximeter. A client of mine underwent cosmetic surgery on his

nose. After the surgeon left the room, he slowly stopped breathing from an overload of pain relievers and sedatives, and no one noticed because the pulse oximeter wasn't working that day. By the time the nurse called 911, his body was cold.)

5. Someone should ask you if you are allergic to any drugs. It may seem like you've been asked this a thousand times, but better too many than not enough. Especially if you are allergic, watch her write down this information.
6. Have you ever had trouble being anesthetized? You may have a "difficult airway"—which means it's hard to put the tube down your throat to assist in breathing while you're paralyzed. Someone needs to ask you about this, and you need to volunteer it if not asked.
7. Does the surgery pose a risk of losing more than half a liter of blood? If so, special precautions need to be undertaken, like starting large-bore intravenous lines and making sure plenty of fluids and blood are available for resuscitation. (In a well-run hospital, you will be asked to donate blood for your own possible transfusions over the weeks leading up to the surgery; this is safer than any stranger's blood.)
8. For most operations, you should receive a dose of preventive antibiotic within one hour before your skin is cut. This is highly effective in preventing wound infections but is inconsistently applied by surgical teams. If it's given too soon, more than an hour or two before the first cut, it will not be as effective. Ask the surgeon ahead of time what the infection prevention routine is, so you can then make sure it's followed. (See Chapter 13 on hospital infections for more on this.)
9. Important X-ray films need to be in the operating room. This is especially true for orthopedic and spinal surgery and cancer surgery. As noted early in this chapter, some horrific cancer tragedies—removal of the healthy organ instead of its diseased mate—would have been prevented if the imaging had been displayed in the OR.

10. A strategy for preventing deadly blood clots in the days and weeks after surgery needs to be decided on before surgery, because the most effective measures work better the sooner they are started. (See Chapter 12 at pages 158–159 for more on blood clot prevention in the hospital.)

As I said, each item on this list needs to be checked off before you are knocked out. If they don't happen, even one of them, or seem to happen in a helter-skelter way, you should consider postponing the surgery. Also remember, you may not be up to enforcing all these items yourself; that's another reason to have an advocate with you at all times, which we'll cover in the next chapter.

The safer-surgery checklist, which includes all of the items described here and more that occur after the patient is asleep, has proven itself in a study conducted among eight hospitals scattered around the world. Before the checklist was implemented, 15 in 1,000 surgery patients died within a month after their operations; after the checklist was in place, 8 in 1,000 died. The injury rate was cut from 110 in 1,000 to 70 in 1,000.[7] Safety has improved not only because of the technical items, like making sure the antibiotic is given and the sponges are counted, but because of at least one significant cultural change: Before the skin is cut, all team members in the operating room are required to pause and introduce themselves to each other by name and role. When this happens, the surgeon is no longer the God of the OR who addresses lower-level staff by barking "Anesthesia!" or "Nurse!"; instead, everyone has a name, and with a name comes respect, better communications, and improved attitudes about safety that translate to saved lives. That these study results were published in January 2009, and not fifty years sooner, only shows how far the health-care system has yet to travel in replacing the old, dangerous, imperial system of surgical treatment with a humane and safe system in which everyone in the OR—and the patient too!—has a valuable role.

Lifesavers:

The Safer-Surgery Checklist

Step Six of our Necessary Nine has been all about finding the right surgeon and maximizing our chances for a healthy outcome. When you use the lists of questions in Chapter 10 for honing in on the right surgeon with the most experience and the best team, you will be pleased to see that a lot of the surgery checklists we have just gone over in Chapter 11 are carried out without much prompting from you or your family. Still, it is important to recognize that bad things happen everywhere in our health-care system, even in the most prestigious institutions, because human beings lack perfection. When doctors and patients use the check-countercheck system from aviation safety, patients can play a valuable part in making sure appropriate things happen. Items where you the patient can make a big difference include getting the most qualified anesthesia provider, making sure your surgeon hasn't confused you with someone else, and getting important safety measures like a pulse oximeter and a preventive antibiotic before surgery.

12

Your Personal Advocate, in the Hospital and Out

Right now, do you have a loved one who is alone in a hospital? Then I have an urgent suggestion: Climb out of the chair and go to their bedside. You can finish reading this chapter when you're there. It's that important for their safety that you or some other smart family member be there for them 24/7.

> *Step Seven:*
> **Have an advocate with you at every significant health-care encounter, especially in the hospital.**

Are you, by any chance, reading this book sitting in a doctor's waiting room, while a family member is behind closed doors getting an examination? Then bookmark this page and go to the exam room. They need you there.

Hospitalized patients lack their usual defenses. All sorts of bad things can happen, and many of them can be prevented by having a family member always present. And even patients who are walking around still need someone with them when they are being examined. That is why Step Seven on our list of the Necessary Nine steps to better health care is "*Have an advocate with you at every significant health-care encounter, especially in the hospital.*"

Here's a checklist of the most common injury-causing events and what you can do to head them off:

- **Falls.** People fall in hospitals all the time, and especially when they're frail and elderly, they can break a hip or some other bone and even die. I cannot tell you how many times I've heard this story: "Mom was so active . . . she still had her mind . . . she was enjoying retirement . . . then she had to be hospitalized for what they said was a routine [fill in the blank], and then she fell one night, and that was the beginning of the end." (In or out of hospitals, falls are the biggest cause of injury, including injury that ends in death, to people over sixty-five; it's been estimated that one in three people over sixty-five can expect to have a fall in any given year.[1]) The most common cause of hospital falls is no surprise: The patient has to go to the bathroom in the middle of the night, in an unfamiliar place, and may have medicines on board that add to confusion and wooziness. They punch the call button. The nurse never seems to come. So they try to negotiate the trip on their own. And the predictable happens. To make sure this never happens, the family member functions as a private-duty nurse. (By the way, if you can afford a private-duty nurse, or even a sitter, by all means, don't let anyone talk you out of it. They are useful in a thousand ways, as I will explain.)
  - But don't try to walk someone to a hospital bathroom without some basic training, especially if the patient is bigger than you. Ask the nurse to show you how it's done.
  - And don't feel obligated to take on these nursing duties if you're scared you might drop Mom or Dad to the floor. If that's so, you can be the squeaking wheel that gets the grease—just add your voice to the patient's voice and it will help win the nurse's attention.

- **Infections.** You can help enforce hygiene. Don't let anyone touch your patient, especially if the patient has any kind of tube stuck in their body or a surgical wound or some other portal of entry for germs, unless you first see them wash their hands in your presence and put on fresh gloves. And don't be fooled by someone who walks in already gloved. What did they touch with those gloves before they got to your patient's room? Likely lots of stuff—other patients' skin, bedrails, monitor buttons, even privacy curtains are all swarming with bugs. Also, don't be fooled by someone who dons a fresh pair of gloves but doesn't first wash their hands. Think about it: As soon as a dirty hand grabs a sterile glove to put it on the other hand, that glove is contaminated. So the only thing that works is washing hands, either with old-fashioned soap and water or an alcohol rub, and then donning gloves. For many more helpful tips on lifesaving infection prevention, see Chapter 13.
- **Bedsores or pressure ulcers.** If your patient is immobile, the hospital needs a regular routine for turning the patient to prevent sores that can turn into gaping wounds that can kill or maim. Find out what the schedule is and enforce it. And you can gently inspect your loved one for early signs of sores—often just a red rash. The two most common areas are the tailbone (sacrum) just above the gluteal cleft, and the heels, because they become pressure points in immobile people. A nickel-size sore can turn into a painful ulcerated wound with breathtaking speed. These ulcers then become infected, and bugs chew up muscle and cause permanent loss of flesh and even death. I've sat across the table from too many family members who, because they didn't know better, didn't look under the bedclothes until the stench of gangrene told them something was terribly wrong. And then it's too late.
- **Medication errors.** These happen every day in even the most advanced hospitals. They especially happen when the hospital

doesn't have a system to catch inevitable human errors that doctors can make when ordering a drug, nurses can make when reading the doctor's scrawl, and pharmacists can make when filling thousands of orders a day. The medical industry also has been slow to adopt standard nomenclature for quantities in drug orders; some doctors write it "1 mg," others "1.0 mg," and if a nurse misses the decimal point, the patient gets 10 mg. You can rest a little easier if you see that the hospital has a bar-code system in which no drug is dispensed to a patient unless the bar code on the patient's wrist matches what's in the nurse's tray. Even that, though, doesn't eliminate all errors. You should at a minimum ask to look at the medications before they're put into your patient's body. Are they the same shape and color as yesterday's medications? If something is new, why? Do you know what each medication is for? How long does your patient need to take the medicine? These are simple but important questions where you can help when your patient is too sick to fend for herself.

- Another secret ally that patients don't use enough—in the hospital or at home—is the pharmacist. Pharmacists have advanced degrees in how drugs work in the body, and especially how drugs interact with each other. Too often, pharmacists are treated like warehouse clerks, when they have so much more to offer. Especially if your loved one is getting medications prescribed by doctors in different specialties, ask the pharmacist to run a check for these drugs' compatibility with each other. (This is the same reason why you should never have prescriptions filled at more than one pharmacy. See Chapter 7 for more on this.)

- **Blood clots in the legs.** The veins deep in our calves are common sites where clots form because blood is stagnant in someone who is not moving their legs. These clots are jellylike snakes that grow bigger and bigger, and when they travel to the veins above the knee, they can eventually reach the heart and plug the arteries feeding blood from the right side of the heart to the lungs, killing the patient with what is known as a pulmonary embolism. Blood clots kill more patients each year than AIDS and breast cancer combined, according to the American College of Chest Physicians.[2] Yet it is now known that nearly all pulmonary embolisms are preventable with a well-thought-out strategy. That includes moving the patient out of bed as soon as possible, applying pressure stockings that massage the calves rhythmically with pulses of compressed air, and administering blood-thinning medicines. So how do you become involved? Ask what the clot prevention strategy is. An amazing percentage of time, especially with patients who are hospitalized for reasons other than surgery, clot prevention is forgotten by providers busy with other work. At the best hospitals now, simple checklists have been implemented to make sure that every patient's risk for clots is measured and appropriately acted on. Dr. Joseph Caprini, a Northwestern University surgeon, developed a two-page form that boils down thousands of pages of medical studies into a simple scoring system for clot risk and a recipe for what each level of risk calls for by way of preventive treatment.[3] Anybody who has had a clot in the past or who has a family history of clots is at especially high risk, another reason to speak up for any hospitalized family member with that background. Fatal clots also can happen outside the hospital. Anyone with a leg immobilized by a cast is at special risk.

Too many of my clients have suffered preventable falls, infections, medication errors, and blood clots in the hospital. But those are only the most obvious injury events that a good advocate can help prevent. Another kind of injury happens when the doctor isn't listening carefully to what the patient is trying to say. Something isn't quite right; the patient doesn't quite know what it is and is inclined to shrug it off. The advocate's voice at this moment can be crucial.

A Physician-Patient's Story: Why Everyone Needs a Patient-Advocate

Patients don't like to complain; no one wants to look ungrateful. So sometimes it's easier for patients who think they're doing 90 percent okay to let the other 10 percent slide. Or the patient will say something, but it just doesn't get through to the busy doctors and overworked nurses. Having your own advocate at your bedside is the best way to nip these misunderstandings in the bud.

Are there any exceptions to who needs a 24/7 advocate with them in the hospital? You might suppose that a patient who is himself a physician could fend for himself. But you would be wrong. A physician client of mine (he asked me to withhold his name) proved that. This physician traveled hundreds of miles from his home, where he was a successful orthopedic surgeon, to Richmond, Virginia, to undergo back surgery with a nationally known spine surgeon. This spine surgeon was using a new artificial disc that seemed promising as a way to relieve the pain from a herniated natural disc but also preserve the mobility in the spine that is the job of our natural discs. Before the artificial discs, surgeons would remove the old disc and fuse together the vertebrae with bone chips and hardware, leaving the back stiff. When my physician client traveled to Richmond for the surgery, his wife accompanied him with their eight-year-old son, but she had her hands full keeping her son in good humor, and came to the hospital only for short visits.

My client knew something was wrong as soon as the anesthesia wore off. His old back pain that had shot down his left leg was gone, but now there was new pain in his right leg that he had never experienced before. He mentioned the pain to the surgeon. Somehow, it didn't sink in that something was seriously wrong. The surgeon gave him extra pain relievers and told him the pain should wear off in a few days or weeks. Three days after the surgery, my client was discharged, and he went to a nearby hotel, and then home, to recuperate. But the pain only worsened. Finally when he couldn't stand it anymore, the physician/patient went to see a neurosurgeon, who promptly had his lower back imaged with dye to make the spinal cord stand out more clearly. Something didn't look right, so the surgeon operated the next day. The surgeon found an olive-size fragment of bone and disc that the first surgeon, while inserting the artificial disc, had somehow dislodged and shoved into the nerve root on the right side of the spine. That explained why the patient had the new, opposite-side pain when he woke up after the surgery. But the two-week delay in removing the fragment had given him a permanent pain syndrome for which he has to take daily narcotic pain relievers.

What might have happened differently? If the patient's wife, herself a nurse, could have been with him in the hospital, another voice of concern, and professional concern at that, would have been added. It wasn't practical for her to be there because of their small son, but if my physician client and his wife had appreciated how crucial it was to have an advocate present, other arrangements could have been made. And then the spine surgeon might not have blown off the patient's concerns about the new pain. The patient also had the kind of human reaction that many patients experience after surgery. You've just placed your life into the hands of a doctor you respect. You've woken alive from the experience. You're grateful for that. It seems almost churlish to complain about new pain. So you mention the pain to your surgeon, but not with the naked emphasis that family members hear. Thus are born misunderstandings that can turn into injuries.

Jim Conway's Story: When Good Communication Is Extra Critical

Any health-care encounter, no matter where it is, can result in someone not hearing what the other person is saying. When the communication is important, that's why you need an extra set of ears, and an extra voice, to help you. Jim Conway told me how he learned this lesson. Just like my physician client, you'd think Jim wouldn't need a helper. Conway is a senior vice president at the Boston-based Institute for Healthcare Improvement. He has a long career as an administrator at prestigious health-care institutions: Children's Hospital in Boston and the Dana-Farber Cancer Institute there. He's spent his life in health care, but he's smart enough to know his own limitations. So when he learned that his diabetes had reached a place where he needed to start daily injections of insulin, his wife, Joanne, went with him to the education session. In the room were Jim, Joanne, a nurse, and an orange. And a needle. Jim thought he heard everything the nurse told him and showed him with the needle puncturing the orange. But the next day, when it was time to inject his skin instead of a piece of fruit, Joanne had to reteach him everything that had gone in one ear and out the other, especially how he needed to push the air out of the syringe before pulling in the insulin. "I guess I thought I heard everything the nurse had told me, but I think I was focusing more on how much was it going to hurt," Jim says now.

When You Cannot Be There in Person

What if you've moved heaven and earth and you just cannot stay at the hospital 24/7 for your hospitalized family member? Here are some options to consider:

- Involve other family members, friends, and neighbors. Set up a bedside rotation. Try to cover as many hours of the day and night as you can.
- Hire a sitter. Sitters are health aides who don't have nursing degrees, but they can provide 99 percent of what's needed: comfort, companionship, help with the little things that drive the bedridden patient insane, and a communication bridge between the hospital staff and the family.
- Pick a lead spokesperson for the family, and give the doctor and nursing staff one cell phone number where that person can always be reached. "If you don't do that," says Thomas Masterson, MD, "and if multiple family members are pulling

the doctor in different directions, you can count on that doctor avoiding you." Dr. Masterson has reason to know; he is a "hospitalist," who does nothing but treat hospitalized patients.

- Negotiate a specific time each day for a telephone briefing with the doctor in charge.

The Daily Talk: What You Must Ask the Doctor in Charge

Whether you can be there in person or have to do it by telephone, you need to have at least one daily communication with the doctor in charge of the patient. But before you have that conversation, first talk to the staff who are spending the most time with your hospitalized loved one: the nurses and therapists. How do they think the patient is doing? What's different today from yesterday?

With your homework done, talk to the doctor. Here are some things that need to be on your checklist of questions.

First and most important, ask, "What is today's plan? What is the specific goal for the day?" Keep a daily checklist of each day's plan, and inquire later to make sure that day's treatment and testing events happened. If there is no daily plan that the doctor can articulate, push for one. Peter Pronovost, MD, the Johns Hopkins critical care doctor who has pioneered patient safety programs around the country, says, "When you manage your own life, you have daily goals, but when people come into the hospital, what I found in my intensive-care rounds is that our daily plans would very often be very vague. Staff members couldn't really say, because they hadn't always thought it through, what they were going to do for each patient each day to get them to the next level of care—out of the ICU or out of the hospital—and how they were going to prevent injuries to the patient. So we developed a simple tool where each day for each patient, we would ask what was needed to get that patient out of intensive care, or out of the hospital, what we were going to do toward that goal, what the patient's greatest safety risks were and what we were going to do about it, and what exactly we were going to do for each organ system. When we implemented that, we dropped length of stay in ICUs in half and we cut medical errors dramatically." So Dr. Pronovost says the patient and the family can help with this by pushing to find out: What will let me go home? Then when the doctor says, it's when you can do A, B, and C, you then find out what's going to happen each day to work toward those goals. These goals are often pretty simple: The patient has to be able to eat, to walk, to move their bowels.

Once the goals are specifically on the table, the rest of the questions fall into place naturally:

- What tests are planned for today and why?
- If tests have been done since the last time you spoke to the doctor, what are the results?
- Are medicines being dropped? New ones added? Why?
- Any specific therapies planned for today? What is the goal?
- How is the patient progressing? Any worries?

Things You Can Help the Doctor Learn

As the bedside advocate, you have a lot of useful information to tell the doctor that otherwise he or she might miss. Here's a short list I picked up from hospitalist Tom Masterson, MD, of things he likes to hear family members alert him to on his rounds:

1. Failure to have a bowel movement.
2. How the patient is doing with walking. Masterson notes, "Remember, the doctor just sees the patient in bed."
3. Swelling of one leg or another. This can be the first sign of a dangerous blood clot. Many doctors, Masterson says, do not take down the sheets in their daily exam.
4. New rashes. A rash can quickly lead to an ulcerated wound if it's at a pressure point.

5. Complaints that might not have been shared with the nurses, such as chest pain, shortness of breath, heartburn, nausea.

The average amount of time a doctor has for each patient on daily rounds is sixteen minutes, says Dr. Masterson, and that includes checking lab and X-ray reports, checking vital signs, reviewing medications, answering nursing questions, examining the patient, and talking to consultants before meeting with you. So the upshot is, says Dr. Masterson, "Chances are, your doctor has already spent too much time on one case, or with another family, and hopes to avoid your questions. But it is vital for the health and well-being for anyone in the hospital to have daily contact with the doctors. So no choice, you have to bother the doctor."

Follow-Up Care: How Your Advocate Can Help at Home

Going home from the hospital is a time of joy and some trepidation for most patients. It's also a time fraught with potential for misunderstandings that can turn into preventable injuries. Says Dr. Pronovost, "So many times patients will be going home and there's ambiguity in what they're supposed to do or what they're supposed to watch out for. You have to be really comfortable leaving the hospital knowing exactly what's supposed to happen next."

The reality is that hospitals don't wait until patients are fully recovered to send them home. Patients are discharged when doctors calculate that the patient can survive at home or a nursing facility or, worse, when an insurance company says benefits are used up. All the care that happened every day in the hospital is now transferred to caregivers at home, like you. So you have to know exactly what is expected. You should insist on a written list of discharge instructions. Most hospitals have a form with fill-in blanks. You might be asked to do any of the following, or more:

- Change bandages and clean a surgical wound.
- Give medications every day.
- Help the patient with walking and other physical exercises. (Remember that all ordinary movements need to be planned. If your patient cannot handle stairs and you live in a walk-up, some solution must be in place before you let the hospital push you out the door. If your patient cannot get in and out of bed without help and you're much smaller than your patient, again, you need a plan before you leave the hospital.)
- Keep an eye on the patient's overall well-being and call the doctor if the patient starts to turn downhill. Obvious things include new pain or new fever. Make sure you know in advance any specific things you are supposed to watch out for.
- Help the patient keep the next appointment at the doctor's office. (This appointment should be made before you leave the hospital.)

Do not let your patient be rolled in her wheelchair meekly and silently out to the curb if you feel uncomfortable taking on any of these tasks. The better option could be a discharge to a rehabilitation facility that has professional staff to ease the transition back to the real world.

What if the patient seems too sick to go home? If the patient seems to you, as the advocate, to be in worse shape, not improving, to be struggling with life-critical functions like breathing, or to have some new problem like a fever or new unexplained pain, you may need to put your foot down. Here is a critical question you should ask, "Are you saying today is the discharge day because in your best medical and nursing judgment, the patient is ready to go home, or is it because the insurance benefits run out today and you don't want to have to fight the insurance bureaucracy for an extension?" Insurance companies set arbitrary limits on hospital stays based on how average patients fare, but you may not fit the average mold. The insurance company likely will relent if the attending doctor sends a strongly worded letter about why more time is needed. But that often doesn't happen unless you, as advocate, ask.

Lifesavers:

Step Seven: What a Patient Advocate (and That Means You) Can Do for Your Loved Ones

Everyone who is sick enough to be in a doctor's office or a hospital bed deserves to have an advocate with them. None of us is at our best when sick; we don't communicate as well, we don't hear as well, and we don't think as well as usual. The advocate becomes our eyes, our ears, and a good part of our brain. Beyond that, the advocate helps us steer clear of the major hazards in every hospital: falls, infections, medication errors, bedsores, and dangerous blood clots. When you become the advocate for a sick family member, you become the go-between between doctor and family, and there are specific questions you should ask (pages 163–164) that will both help the doctors do their job and also keep anxious family members calm. You want to prevent decisional drift and keep everyone focused on specific goals for getting your patient back into the healthy mainstream. When you take the patient home, another list of questions (page 166) needs to be answered first so that the home care gets done safely and thoroughly. Don't let anyone, especially an insurance bureaucrat, force you to leave the hospital if your patient seems too sick.

13

The Scandal of Infections in Hospitals and Other Health-Care Facilities, and What You Can Do

You may think of hospitals as sterile, healthy environments. They actually can be—especially in the patient rooms—filthy and dangerous places for catching horrible bugs that can kill. I have devoted an entire chapter to what I call the scandal of infections in hospitals, clinics, and other care facilities, because you need to know how bad it is out there, and then you will appreciate why you need to take some fairly drastic measures to protect yourself and your loved ones in the hospital. We have already met some of the major hazards of hospitals in Chapter 12. Now we will wade more deeply into the quagmire, as we focus on Step Eight of our Necessary Nine, starting with this chapter: *Learn how to steer clear of the major hazards of hospitals and how to find hospitals that work to maximize*

> *Step Eight:*
> **Learn how to steer clear of the major hazards of hospitals and how to find hospitals that work to maximize your safety.**

your safety. In this chapter, we will see some of the ways to avoid infection in hospitals, and then the next chapter will probe more generally into the difficult task of finding all-around quality hospitals.

To appreciate the true scandal of hospital infections, consider some history. Medicine first began to understand that lives could be saved by doctors washing their hands in 1846, in Vienna, Austria. Ignaz Semmelweis, a cranky and compulsive obstetrician, counted deaths from what was then called childbed fever, which mothers contracted shortly after giving birth. He noticed that at one clinic, as many as three in ten mothers were dying, but at another, hardly any did. The deliveries at the clinic with the high death rate were all done by physicians, while the clinic with few deaths was run by midwives. Semmelweis observed that the doctors attending the more prosperous mothers in the (not coincidentally named) First Clinic would arrive in the obstetric unit directly from the autopsy suite, and even though they washed their hands with soap and water, their hands still carried a foul odor. He thought "cadaverous particles" were carried on the doctors' hands. Semmelweis insisted that all the physicians and medical students wash their hands with a chlorine solution between every patient. The deaths of mothers quickly plummeted. But the idea that doctors needed to wash their hands offended many of his colleagues, who saw themselves as gentlemen in no need of special hygienic practices. Moreover, the impressive statistics from Semmelweis could not withstand the then current medical received wisdom, which held, with the ancient Greeks, that the body's four humors caused all disease, not some microscopic particles that no one had ever seen. Semmelweis was ridiculed, rejected, and removed from the faculty of his hospital. He died in an insane asylum a few weeks after his forty-seventh birthday, in 1865. Within twenty years, the work of Louis Pasteur, Joseph Lister, and Robert Koch produced the germ theory of disease, and Semmelweis was belatedly recognized as a visionary.

A parallel story occurred in America around the same time. Oliver Wendell Holmes, whose son became the famous Supreme Court justice of the same name, published a book proposing that hand washing would prevent the spread of deadly disease. "In my own family," he wrote, "I had rather that those I esteemed the most should be delivered unaided, in a stable, by the mangerside, than that they should receive the best help, in the fairest apartment, but exposed to the vapors of this pitiless disease." Holmes, too, was ridiculed. Charles Meigs, a well-known obstetrician, sniffed, "Doctors are gentlemen, and gentlemen's hands are clean."

Fast-forward to 2002. Yet another effort is mounted to coax doctors and nurses to clean their hands before touching patients. A task force of leaders from major infectious disease societies issues a report called "Guideline for Hand Hygiene in Health-Care Settings."[1] The report writers feel compelled to document their recommendations with no fewer than 423 footnotes. They note that theirs is the latest in a series of guidelines issued by the U.S. Public Health Service and other health agencies. Other landmark dates came and went in 1961, 1975, 1985, 1988, and 1995. Despite all the guidelines and their adoption by most but not all hospitals, the 2002 report dryly observes, "Adherence of health-care workers to recommended hand hygiene procedures has remained poor."[2] The least likely to use good practices, they write, are male physicians; the most likely to comply are nurses. The places in the hospital with the lowest compliance with good hand hygiene are intensive care units, where the patients are the sickest and most vulnerable to infection.[3]

How Many Joan Dalys?

At age sixty-three, in excellent health except for well-controlled adult-onset diabetes, Joan Daly slipped on ice outside a restaurant and broke her shoulder in January 2004. She underwent surgery at the prestigious Hospital for Joint Diseases in New York City. Just before discharge, her daughter Maureen Daly watched as a doctor, a senior resident (near the end of his training years), changed her mother's dressings—with bare, unwashed hands. Five days later, Joan developed intense pain. When the dressing was removed, a foul odor filled the room, and Maureen saw "this greenish fluid coming out of her arm, oozing and oozing." Joan Sullivan Daly, daughter of a Brooklyn pub owner, who almost became a nun before a whirlwind courtship with the eldest son of family friends, died months later of MRSA, a drug-resistant bacterial infection. To see her mother die of a preventable infection was unbearable to Maureen, her sister, Marie, and their father, Danny. Now, Maureen and other family members regularly volunteer at the advocacy group Committee to Reduce Infection Deaths (RID) in an effort to get the word out.

Many more examples of real people who were killed or maimed by hospital-acquired infections are collected at the Web site of another advocacy group, Consumers Union, which is pushing states to require hospitals to publicly report their infection rates. [4]

How many Joan Daly's are there in the United States? Every year, 100,000 or more patients die of preventable hospital-acquired infections—more deaths than AIDS, breast cancer, and auto accidents combined. (That's on top of the 100,000 deaths that were estimated by the landmark 1999 study that we talked about in the Introduction.) Some 2 million patients come down with infections in the hospital and have to undergo costly and debilitating treatments, sometimes losing limbs and teetering for months on the brink of death. These numbers come from the Committee to Reduce Infection Deaths. RID's tireless president, Betsy McCaughey, says the rates may actually be much higher, since the government does such a spotty job of tracking infections in hospitals.[5]

The scandal of hospital infections deepens still further. It's almost as if an evil scientist were conducting an experiment. Take a group of people who are at highest risk of infections because their bodies' natural resistance has been worn down by disease and injury. Mix them all together so people who carry deadly infectious agents share rooms with uncontaminated people. Then circulate among these patients a group of workers who touch every patient, one after the other, but who follow basic rules about hand washing and glove wearing less than half the time.[6] Then, to make things worse still, clean the rooms of these infected patients so that the floors are mopped, and the rooms look superficially clean, but all the surfaces touched by the infected patients and by the contaminated, unwashed hands of the hospital workers—the call buttons, bed rails, tray tables, IV pump switches, bathroom faucets, privacy curtains—remain uncleaned and teeming with germs.[7] That is a recipe for the disaster we have in American hospitals today.

Of course, no evil scientist planned it this way; the road to hell, in this case, is paved with a thousand excuses: Hand cleaners irritate the skin; the dispenser is empty; the patient needs me first; time is short; I forgot. Exactly the kind of situation where the government should step in with firm rules, instead of timid guidelines, but so far, the lead federal agency, the Centers for Disease Control and Prevention, has taken a voluntaristic approach whose failures are hidden by the secrecy of its data. But I'm getting ahead of the story.

The Evolution of MRSA—and How to Stop It

This disaster was slow in the building. Within a few years after penicillin was discovered by Alexander Fleming in 1943, nearly any bacterial infection could be cured with a liberal dose of antibiotics. But the bugs fought back. One very common target for antibiotics was *Staphylococcus aureus*, a bug that lives harmlessly on the skin and in the nostrils of up to one-third of Americans, but which can cause nasty infections once it gets inside the body. This is the very bug that Fleming proved with his petri dish could be killed by the fungus whose active ingredient was penicillin. MRSA—which stands for methicillin-resistant *Staphylococcus aureus*—is the staph bug's second evolutionary wave of response to penicillin and other antibiotics. The first was to develop an enzyme that broke down penicillin. Bacteriologists responded by developing drugs like methicillin, which resisted the enzyme's attack. Then MRSA came along, first detected in a tiny number of cases in Great Britain in the early 1960s, now worldwide. MRSA is a stubborn bug that can live for hours on hospital-room surfaces and fabrics like staff uniforms. So it's easily carried from one patient to another.

The good news is that the cures for this epidemic disease are already at hand:

- rigorous hand washing (with soap and water or an alcohol gel) and wearing gloves before touching the patient, and especially before invading the patient's body with any tube or needle of any kind;
- screening of all new patients with nasal swabs and isolating patients who carry drug-resistant germs in special rooms;
- changing uniforms every shift, with new gowns or disposable plastic aprons used for any contact with infected patients, or patients who are carriers but not themselves infected (the doctor's white coat, which often isn't cleaned for weeks on end, is a notorious carrier of germs);
- using disposable equipment for anything that might touch more than one patient—such as disposable liners for blood pressure cuffs, EKG leads, etc.;
- "soak and wait" cleaning of all surfaces in patient rooms that any patient or staff might come in contact with (waiting a minute or two before wiping off disinfectant); and
- administering a dose of an antibiotic one to two hours before any surgical patient is cut open.

These precautions have been proven, through widespread use in Denmark, Holland, and Finland, to cut hospital-acquired infection rates to next to nothing. Unfortunately, they have not been widely adopted in the United States, aside from a few hospitals like the Veterans Administration system—pioneered by its hospital in Pittsburgh.[8] But the trend is in the right direction. We are in the midst of a sea change, from the old complacency—based on the wrong but persistent idea that infections are just one of those things that happen in hospitals, and that's why patients should go home as soon as they can—to the new enthusiasm for making sure that nobody leaves the hospital worse off than they came in, by using rigorous hygiene practices. Until these practices become widespread, however, hospitals are still very dangerous places, and patients need to look carefully to find those that take prevention of infection seriously.

Protecting Yourself from Hospital Infections

Twenty-two states now require public reporting of infection rates, so patients can make their own comparisons.[9] But of those twenty-two, only three so far—Florida, Pennsylvania, and Missouri—have issued public report cards on their hospitals. More will follow soon. Consumers Union is pushing Congress to make this a uniform national requirement.

What you can get, in the meantime, is data on how hard the hospitals try. One benchmark is the hospital's percent of surgical patients who receive an appropriate preventative antibiotic within an hour before surgery. This is the number-one most effective way to prevent what can be deadly infections of the surgical wound. There's a huge variation in how consistently patients receive this proven treatment. According to a study by Consumers Union, the lowest-rated hospitals in Virginia gave appropriately timed antibiotics to about one in four surgical patients, while the best hospitals in the state had an almost perfect 97 percent record.[10]

While we wait to get enough information so we can vote with our feet and shun the hospitals with bad infection rates, the question is, what do we as patients do in the meantime?

As a patient, you could go crazy trying to make sure you aren't infected. And you could drive your caregivers crazy too, as you shriek at them, "Don't touch me until you've washed your hands!" There is no ideal way to protect yourself and remain the cheerful, compliant patient whom many patients think they need to be so the nurses treat them gently and don't withhold treatments.

But consider this simple fact: A bug like MRSA can rampage through your body once it gets inside, defeating most of the antibiotics that doctors throw at it, but when it's on the outside, lurking on the bedrail, or the glove of the nurse taking your temperature, any cleaner with alcohol in it will kill it. Windex works. So does Mister Clean. So for hands, use any of the alcohol-based hand sanitizers that many hospitals are finally starting to put in all patient rooms.

What's a Patient to Do?

When you're in a new environment like a hospital room, you don't know what germs the last patient had, or how effectively the room was scrubbed after the patient left. You don't know what germs that nice nurse was just exposed to before she arrived to do her first evaluation of you. What's a patient to do? Here is patient-advocate Betsy McCaughey's advice.

1. *Enforce hand washing for everyone immediately before they touch you.* This is essential but not easy. Dr. McCaughey says, "Fortunately hospitals are making it easier and easier to speak up; you will see signs everywhere about hand washing and urging patients to speak up." Know that if the caregiver touches with their hands *any surface* in your room, including the privacy curtain, after they have washed and gloved their hands, they have potentially recontaminated themselves and need to start again.
2. *Watch your tone of voice.* The old maxim that you catch more bears with honey than with vinegar works with nurses, too. "I know you're working very hard, but I'm very worried about these germs, and would you please . . ." McCaughey also notes what she tells patients who are timid because of "white coat syndrome." "I tell them to remember how dirty that white coat is. Studies show that 65 percent admit they change their white lab coat less than once a week." The doctor's tie, which dangles over the patient, also is another proven avenue for infection to spread.
3. *Don't be lulled into complacency by gloves alone.* If a health-care worker goes from patient to patient with the same pair of

gloves on, the only person protected is the worker herself, because germs are passed on just as effectively from the surface of gloves as from bare hands. And even if they don a new pair of gloves in front of you, if they haven't washed their hands first, they are contaminating the gloves in the process of putting them on with dirty hands.

4. *Read and take with you to the hospital the list that the Committee to Reduce Infection Deaths put together, called Fifteen Steps You Can Take to Reduce Your Risk of a Hospital Infection.* I've reprinted the list as an appendix with Dr. McCaughey's permission (see pages 267–269). The list is an empowering tool. As Dr. McCaughey says, "When patients and families have the fifteen steps as a written brochure, it gives them much more clout; they can say, 'Look, this brochure is telling me to say this to you.' So this makes it less personal."
5. *When you arrive in your hospital room, assume it's contaminated and have a good cleaning done by your advocate.*[11] Here's how Dr. McCaughey copes when she knows a family member or friend is being admitted to the hospital: "I discreetly go in with a cleaner in my purse and wipe all the surfaces. Almost any detergent will kill these bugs. The trick is to leave it on long enough. You need to cover the surface with detergent for three minutes. Just spray it and let it sit. It's the length of time that's important, rather than the ingredients. Then wipe it off."

That last tip applies to tough bugs like MRSA, its cousin VISA, and another superbug called VRE (vancomycin-resistant *Enterococcus*). Further action is needed for another superbug called *Clostridium difficile* ("*C. diff.*" in hospital jargon). *C. diff.* causes terrible watery diarrhea that can be fatal if the patient is already weak. It's harder to kill because it lives in hard-to-penetrate spores, so you either have to use bleach to kill it, or, says Dr. McCaughey, use an individual disposable wipe on each separate surface and wipe the spores away and into the trash can. It's important not to use the same wipe on more than one surface, because then you're just pushing around the *C. diff.* spores.

6. *Wash with a chlorhexidine-based soap before you go to the hospital.* Another thing you can do to reduce your risk of postoperative infections of the surgical site (the place where the surgeon's knife enters your skin) by up to two-thirds is to bathe daily, for three to five days before the surgery, with a 4 percent chlorhexidine soap like Hibiclens. That kills the bugs on your skin that might be dangerous if they had a chance to sneak in through the surgical wound.

See the appendix on pages 267–269 for more lifesaving tips to reduce your risk of a hospital-acquired infection. I know that some of you are still hesitant, so let's hear another word from Joan Daly's daughter Maureen, a volunteer at RID: "With my work at RID, I tell patients every day that they and their families are the best advocates. I encourage them to speak up about any condition or concern they have. Most especially, I remind them to insist that they see all medical professionals wash and glove hands in front of them. I am often asked, 'Won't I offend them or insult them?' My response is, 'Your life depends on this.' I share the biggest regret of my life with them. That regret is allowing the physician to change Mom's dressings without gloving or washing his hands. I only wish I had done something to stop this. I invite people to see themselves as consumers of health-care services, rather than patients. We are 'hiring' a professional to perform a service that we can not do ourselves, we put our trust in them to 'do no harm.' When we engage a realtor, we ask many questions. No one would ever say, 'Sell my house, and let me know what you sold it for.' The health-care consumer has many choices in hiring which hospitals and physicians. The consumer should ask questions about any concern they have prior to a hospital admission. If their concerns are not met, I encourage them to find a new provider."

Another Deadly but Preventable Hospital Infection

Here is another kind of hospital infection you need to know about, because it's so deadly yet so preventable, and you won't be able to protect yourself once you are lying in the hospital. I'm talking about bloodstream infections caused by catheters inserted into either a large artery or a large vein—known in the business as "central lines," which deliver large quantities of drugs, nutrients, and other lifesaving material, and which also deliver monitors of blood pressure to the heart itself. If you need one of these central-line catheters, you are one sick puppy, and likely are in an intensive-care unit, where use of central lines is extremely common. It used to be that infections of the blood caused by these central lines were accepted as unpreventable, even though anywhere from one in ten to four in ten patients who developed these infections died. Pioneering research by one of the true heroes of hospital quality, Dr. Peter Pronovost of Johns Hopkins, has proven that these once-fatal infections can nearly always be prevented. How? By use of a simple checklist to make sure that hygienic practices are rigorously followed when central lines are inserted. When workers insert one of these sterile lines, they have to clean the skin with chlorhexidine first, then use full barrier precautions like you would see in an operating room—masks, gowns, gloves, and sterile drapes. One key feature that makes the program work is that any caregiver on the team—typically, a nurse—is empowered to call a halt to the insertion of the central line if he or she observes any deviation from the standard checklist.

Other Health-Care Facilities: Even Scarier

Don't think you can avoid unnecessary infections by just staying out of hospitals and getting all your care in outpatient clinics or surgery centers. It's a jungle out there. In fact, repeated epidemics of life-threatening infections have occurred in outpatient clinics that would be unimaginable in any hospital because the clinics violated basic injection practices that every hospital nurse learns in the first week on the job.

A group of pain clinics in New York City, another pain center in Norman, Oklahoma, a pain clinic in Nassau County, on Long Island, New York, an endoscopy clinic in Las Vegas, Nevada, and a cancer chemotherapy clinic in Fremont, Nebraska, all shared the dubious distinction in the early 2000s of infecting dozens of their patients with hepatitis B and hepatitis C.[12] Both viruses can cause debilitating, even fatal liver damage. How did they do it? At the Long Island clinics, all run by an anesthesiologist named Harvey Finkelstein, multiple-dose anesthetic vials were used first on an infected patient, then used again on others, spreading infection to at least four patients. At the Nevada surgery center, a similar event happened with anesthetic vials, and so, too, at the Oklahoma pain clinic. The anesthetists didn't realize that if they changed needles between patients, but then reused a contaminated syringe (the tube that holds the medicine), infection could easily spread. More than one hundred patients ultimately were found to have been infected with hepatitis B or C in the Oklahoma clinic alone.

At the Nebraska clinic, a nurse used a syringe to draw blood, then used the same syringe to flush out an IV line with saline, then reused the 500 cc saline bag on other patients. CDC investigators documented that ninety-nine patients were infected with hepatitis C. The clinic had no active infection-control program. What the nurse did was a gross violation of aseptic technique, but she didn't know better. The nurse and the oncologist supervisor had their licenses revoked.

The CDC concluded that all of these cases were entirely preventable with standard precautions and aseptic technique. How did the CDC respond? With a new, nonmandatory "guideline" of course![13] The guideline repeated standard wisdom that had been lost somehow in these outpatient settings. For example, if a nurse injects one patient from a syringe, she cannot inject another patient with the same syringe, even if she changes the needle, and even if she didn't "pull back" on the plunger before injecting the first patient. Anybody who's ever shared a bottle of Coke with a friend knows that "backwash" means you're sharing germs no matter how carefully you wipe off the rim. It's a little more serious when you're introducing the shared stuff into the bloodstream.

What to Watch for When You're Being Injected

Whenever you're injected with medication, look to see that the health-care worker is using

1. a new vial of medicine that hasn't been used on other patients,
2. a new sterile syringe, and
3. a new sterile needle attached to the syringe.

You can tell it's new by all the packaging they have to rip open. Anything less than all three of those will subject you to a huge risk of contracting a life-threatening infection.[14]

In New York, Dr. Finkelstein stopped using the same syringe with multiple patients after state health officials pointed out the error, so the state's medical licensing authorities decided no discipline was warranted. The state did pass a new law in 2008 to give doctors under investigation for improper care just one day to turn over patient records.[15] The same law requires state licensing authorities to regularly review malpractice settlements for any disquieting patterns. It turns out that Finkelstein had accumulated ten malpractice settlements in a decade.[16] That puts him way out on the fringe. When I've sued doctors, I could count on one hand those who had more than two or three prior lawsuits.

It's fashionable in patient-safety research to talk about system failures. Hospitals don't always have enough antiseptic dispensers available. They don't always teach their staff how long to rub their hands together and what skin surfaces are most important to cover. They overwork the staff and don't give them time to do the basic standard procedures. But what happens when the institutions get it right, but the individuals still don't follow through? *What is the excuse?* Dr. Semmelweis is asking. The *New England Journal of Medicine* published an article on this topic in 2006. It had the evocative title, "System Failure Versus Personal Accountability—the Case for Clean Hands." The author, Donald Goldmann, concluded, "When a doctor or nurse can reduce the spread of antibiotic-resistant bacteria by practicing simple hand hygiene, accountability should matter. True, the hospital and its leaders are accountable for establishing a system in which caregivers have the knowledge, competence, time, and tools to practice perfect hygiene. But each caregiver has the duty to perform hand hygiene—perfectly and every time. When this widely accepted, straightforward standard of care is violated, we cannot continue to blame the system."[17]

Dr. Semmelweis couldn't have said it better.

The Big Picture: Let's Think About Safety Reform

Before we leave the subject of hospital-acquired infections, I want to spend another minute pursuing my not-so-hidden subagenda in this book: persuading you about the urgency of major reform in the health-care system—more carrots, more sticks—to make sure recognized lifesaving practices happen every time. My example du jour is surgical site infections. These are the second most common hospital-acquired infections after those in the urinary tract. If you acquire one, you will likely spend time in an ICU, you will be five times more likely than an uninfected patient to need to be readmitted to the hospital, and you will be twice as likely to die. No one knows exactly how many patients contract these, because there is no mandated central clearinghouse of statistics, but various studies say that in two to fifteen of every one hundred surgical procedures, the patient winds up with a surgical site infection. If we conservatively estimated the rate at four in one hundred, that would be a little under a million patients a year.[18] No matter how you slice the numbers, it's a huge problem. But there's a simple answer: A dose of prophylactic antibiotics given within two hours (or better, one hour) before surgery reduces the infection rate to well under 1 percent. It's well documented that if the antibiotics aren't given until after the skin is cut, the rate of infections goes way up. Too soon, before the magic one- to two-hour window, and infection rates also go up. And so it's now considered standard practice to give these antibiotics for almost every kind of surgery. How often does it happen? A major national survey in 2005 found that barely more than *half* of the patients got the dose of antibiotics they were supposed to receive within an hour before the first cut.[19] That is why in Chapter 11, our checklist for safe surgery included having you, the patient, or your advocate, make sure you receive the antibiotic, since there is about a fifty-fifty chance it will not be administered unless you speak up.

Why don't surgical patients receive these drugs nearly every time, the way they are supposed to? Canadian researchers did in-depth interviews of surgeons, anesthesiologists, and nurses at two major hospitals, and found five main reasons: low priority, inconvenience, "workflow," communication, and what they delicately called role perception. Translation: "Not my job."[20]

Patients could easily say it's not their job, either. They're not being paid to give the medicine. But until a better system of accountability is in place, patients are the ones who do pay when it doesn't happen.

Health-care finance reform has been on the agenda of Congress and various state legislatures off and on since the early 1990s. Finance reform and safety reform go hand in hand. If we ever implement a single-payer system, like Medicare for all, it will be a lot easier to implement safety reforms, since the payer will have the clout to enforce rules for quality care. Anyone who has experienced health care in Europe, or in the U.S. Veterans Administration, knows that "socialized medicine," while not perfect, actually can deliver higher-quality, lower-cost medicine day in and day out than the free enterprise, insurance-based system we have. And anyone who learns that Medicare's administrative costs total three cents of every dollar in its budget, whereas private health insurers keep twenty-five to thirty cents of every premium dollar for administrative costs and profit, knows that something drastic needs to happen. If health-care reform consists only in making insurance companies cover more people, without any safety reform, we will ensure that the safety and quality mess gets worse; it will just be spread around to more people. What we the patients should push for, in my view, are these reforms:

- Universal access to health care, paid by the government. This is the way it works in virtually every other civilized country. Many thoughtful doctors favor such a program because it would cut out the tremendous waste that private insurers inflict on our current nonsystem, but would leave clinical decisions to patients and their doctors. The group Physicians for a National Health Program has details on its Web site.[21]
- Financial accountability for health-care providers who inflict injury on patients. The nasty secret of our current system is that when a patient suffers a fall, or a pressure ulcer, or an operative wound infection, or some other preventable injury, hospitals *make more money*, because they are paid to treat both the patient's original condition and the new injury. Medicare started a pilot project in 2008 to force hospitals to swallow the cost of treating some of the injuries they have caused. This needs to be a universal rule, and it should apply to individual providers and not only institutions.
- Full disclosure to the public of all injury events at every hospital, clinic, surgery center, and nursing home. These numbers are collected now only on a voluntary and secret basis—although some progressive states have mandated disclosure to a state health agency. The current patchwork system makes it hard for patients to find the best hospitals, as I explain in more detail in the next chapter.
- Regular audits of quality-of-care measures, and public access to results. We have already seen how surveys have documented the American "half-not" system—that on average American

patients receive only about half of the care recommended by expert consensus and authoritative studies of what kinds of care give the longest, healthiest lives. (See Chapter 1, pages 4–6.) These research surveys need to be taken to the next level: routine audits of doctors' offices, clinics, and hospitals on quality of care. Medicare has started to do this for hospitals, as we will discuss in the next chapter, but the audits cover only a short list of diseases. In the meantime, in Chapter 16, I discuss how patients can audit their own care to make sure they're getting the right stuff.

- Better conflict-of-interest rules. We've talked about the drug companies in Chapter 7, and more about conflicts of interest in Chapter 9. Patients have a right to receive recommendations for their care that are not tainted by profit concerns. At a minimum, patients should be able to find out what companies have paid money to their doctors.

Reform along these lines will not stop all injuries and errors, but it would go a long way toward improving quality of care for everyone and giving patients the information we need so we can give our health-care business to those who are working the hardest to keep us safe.

Livesavers:

Wash Your Hands!

A little knowledge goes a long way toward preventing tragedy. Just knowing how many bugs lurk in health-care facilities—and how easy they are to fight off with rigorous sanitation practices—can arm us to insist on basic precautions when germ-laden health-care workers approach our sick family members. Wash your hands! Put on the gloves in our presence! We don't want to bark at nurses and doctors, but we do need to see these precautions taken. Our eyes can be our allies, too, in other situations with high risk of infection transmission, when "central lines" are being placed in a family member in the ICU, when we receive an injection in any health-care setting, when the clock is ticking toward a surgical procedure and a preventive antibiotic should be administered. In each setting, knowing the simple practices that health-care workers are supposed to follow can alert us to make sure it happens. Still, because this involves a lot more work than any patient or patient's family should have to do, we need to campaign for public accountability for the germ spreaders. Let there be a hall of shame for all patients to see, and then we can vote on where we want to be treated—with our feet.

14

Looking for the Best Hospital: A Frustrating Journey with Some Hope

We ought to be able to pick our hospitals with at least as much intelligence as we use to find a good restaurant. Imagine being able to pick up a hospital review that answers three basic questions:

- How satisfied are patients at this hospital with their care?
- How well does the hospital comply with proven safety and quality strategies?
- How many patients die or suffer an injury that should not have happened?

The good news is that government and private organizations have started to make this vital information available to all of us. The bad news is that the information now available is fragmented, spotty, complicated, and overly reliant on voluntary self-reporting by hospitals. Still, what's being reported by these infant systems is intriguing, sometimes surprising, and definitely worth knowing about if you have any say over where you or a loved one will be next hospitalized.

A Search for Information: Then and Now

Medicare, the government finance system for medical care for patients sixty-five and older, has been gathering data for a long time on basic things like how many people live and die with a given disease, or after a certain kind of surgery. Medicare knows this information for every hospital and every doctor. In the late 1970s, when I was a medical reporter at the *Miami Herald*, I found out that the private agencies that took our tax dollars to collect and organize this data for Medicare (these outfits are now officially called Quality Improvement Organizations) could track each surgeon's volume of cases, complication rates, and death rates. At that time, a dozen hospitals in Miami did lucrative coronary-bypass surgeries, way too many hospitals to generate enough volume for each surgeon to be really proficient and keep his or her patients alive. So the data would have been fascinating. But it turned out the numbers were shrouded in secrecy. So that was one story I never wrote.

Flash-forward to 2008. Medicare now, finally, has a Web site that makes public some of the information Medicare knows. It doesn't list individual doctors, but it does give information for specific hospitals. I looked up death rates at http://www.hospitalcompare.hhs.gov. Medicare puts on the Web site the hospital-mortality information for only two conditions: heart attack and congestive heart failure (that's when the heart, weakened by disease, loses the ability to pump efficiently). For any one hospital, you do not see actual numbers; instead you are told if its death rate fits into one of three categories: average, significantly above average, or significantly below average.

At least it's a start. But here's the real disappointment. Nearly all hospitals in the United States are average, according to Medicare. Of the 4,477 hospitals about which the government has collected the thirty-day death rates after treatment for heart attack,[1] 4,453 have death rates no different than the U.S. national rate of 16 percent. Only seventeen hospitals are better than the U.S. national rate, and only seven are worse.[2] That's a lot of average-ness!

What's going on here? The footnotes on the Hospital Compare Web site say that the government kicks a hospital out of the average group only if the statistics show a 95 percent certainty that the hospital's difference is not due to chance or to having a different mix of patients. That's called risk adjustment; the idea is to massage the statistics so that hospitals don't look artificially good just because they treat a healthier population and vice versa. Statisticians need to make this adjustment to be fair, but where they draw the line between average and below average is controversial. I asked an independent expert in measuring hospital death rates what he thought. Dr. Ashish Jha, an assistant professor at the Harvard School of Public Health, says Medicare chose "an incredibly conservative risk adjustment scheme, too conservative, I think." In August 2008, in response to critics like Dr. Jha, Medicare finally started putting the actual death numbers on its Hospital Compare Web site, although they are well hidden. (Look for the discussion of mortality graphs and then click on View Graph.) But even though you can now see actual numbers, Medicare still applies a formula that results in a statistical range in which nearly all hospitals fall into the average group.

Bottom line: Meaningful death rates are not available from the major government collector of that information, which would rather keep consumers in the dark than offend some of its powerful hospital constituents.

A commercial company, HealthGrades Inc., has stepped into the void. On its Web site, http://www.healthgrades.com, you can find how hospitals fare on survival and avoiding complications for a variety of medical and surgical conditions. Ironically, most of its data comes from the same Medicare database where Hospital Compare says that nearly all hospitals are average—except that HealthGrades includes only 70 percent in the average category and gives ratings above average for 15 percent of hospitals and below average for another 15 percent.

The problem is that HealthGrades doesn't tell independent experts how it manages to find 15 percent best and 15 percent worst among American hospitals, where Medicare could find far less than 1 percent best and worst from the same information. So experts like Harvard's Dr. Jha are skeptical of the usefulness of HealthGrades's death and complication rates.

I looked up the HealthGrades report for what is universally recognized as one of the nation's top hospitals, Johns Hopkins in Baltimore. *U.S. News & World Report* regularly crowns Hopkins number one in its annual ratings, which are based on a complex formula that includes reputation, death rates, and other factors. But according to HealthGrades, Hopkins had better than average survival and complication rates for just a few conditions: chronic obstructive lung disease, heart failure, pancreatitis, and stroke. Hopkins rated worse than average in appendectomy, spinal fusion, heart balloon and stent procedures, heart attack, hip fracture, maternity care, newborn survival, sepsis (blood infection), and valve-replacement surgery. It was average in fifteen other areas. That means Hopkins is far more mediocre than its reputation suggests, or that the HealthGrades ratings deserve some skepticism. Maybe a little of both. My conclusion is that comparing hospitals by outcomes—death and injury rates—is not quite ready for prime time.

Other Ways to Compare Hospitals

Let's talk about two other ways to compare hospitals: how well they do on safety and quality "process" measures, and patient satisfaction. First, the process measures.

I discuss in other chapters some of the proven lifesaving tactics that researchers know hospitals should be doing. For example,

- heart-attack victims will live longer if, as soon as possible after hitting the emergency room, they receive aspirin and a beta-blocker drug to minimize damage to the heart muscle (Chapter 16); and

- patients catch far fewer infections in the hospital if the hospital adheres to a strict hygiene policy, gives patients a preventive dose of antibiotics just before surgery, and isolates carriers of antibiotic-resistant bugs (Chapters 11 and 13).

Another simple step, and an easily measurable one, is full, 24/7 staffing of intensive care units by intensive-care specialists (also called intensivists or critical-care specialists). When intensive care is provided by doctors who try to juggle visits to the ICU with their other patient-care duties, the ICU patients can suffer.

Two Web sites are starting to publicize how well individual hospitals comply with some of these safety and quality strategies.

Medicare's Hospital Compare Web Site

On the Medicare Web site, you can find specific quality scores in the following areas (all listings are for the percent of patients in the hospital's overall self-reporting who received one or more specific interventions in each category):

- preventive antibiotics for surgery patients,
- treatment to prevent blood clots in surgery patients,
- heart attack,
- pneumonia, and
- heart failure.

On the Hospital Compare Web site, you can set up a side-by-side comparison with as many as three hospitals. You will likely find that most hospitals score over 90 percent compliance on each of the measures. For example, I compared Yale–New Haven Hospital in Connecticut with two lesser-known nearby hospitals but which have good local reputations: Griffin Hospital in Derby, Connecticut, and St. Vincent's Medical Center in Bridgeport, Connecticut. The percent of heart-attack patients who got a beta-blocker drug at discharge was 98 percent at Griffin, 99 percent at St. Vincent's, and 98 percent at Yale–New Haven. Yale scored a little worse than its lesser-known brethren in blood clot prevention, surgery antibiotics, and heart failure discharge instructions.

Why do most hospitals score close to each other on these quality "process" measures? I can think of two possibilities:

- Because Medicare gave hospitals plenty of warning that they would be graded on these measures, something could be going on like what happens with schools in No Child Left Behind—the hospitals "teach to the test" and make sure their staffs do well with whatever Medicare happens to be measuring, even if they don't do so well on the quality measures that outsiders don't examine closely.
- Or it could be that hospitals are generally getting a lot better in their safety and quality.

When I talked to health-care safety experts, the takeaway message was mixed: They hope hospitals are genuinely improving in their overall quality and safety practices but aren't sure if the evidence really bears it out. And the bottom line—whether these "process" improvements translate into measurable reductions in preventable deaths and injuries—just isn't known yet, because deaths and injures are still sketchily measured and spottily reported.

The Leapfrog Group

The Leapfrog Group is a consortium of sixty-five employers and agencies that buy health care for more than 34 million Americans. Leapfrog was started in 2000 to try to coax better care voluntarily out of hospitals by publicizing how well hospitals comply with a lot of quality measures that aren't covered on Medicare's Hospital Compare Web site. Its coverage is not nearly as comprehensive as Medicare; only about 1,300 hospitals of the nation's 5,400 hospitals were participating in Leapfrog's annual survey as of 2008, but those are concentrated in big metropolitan areas, so more than half the U.S. population can find a Leapfrog-surveyed hospital nearby.

Leapfrog's quality measures so far include

- computerized order-entry systems for medications and tests, which can dramatically cut medication errors in wrong drug or wrong dose;
- ICU staffing by full-time intensivists;
- adherence to a list of twenty-seven safety standards from the National Quality Forum, a respected independent group that works to come up with consensus lists of good and bad safety practices throughout medical care (Leapfrog surveys on thirteen of the standards);
- how hospitals handle injuries that experts agree should never happen (burns, falls, deep pressure ulcers, and others; see Appendix 261, which lists these). Leapfrog asks hospitals to voluntarily agree to do four things: Apologize to the patient, report the event to a public health agency, analyze its root cause, and waive costs related to the event.

So far, about 700 of Leapfrog's 1,300 targeted hospitals have agreed to implement this policy.[3] Leapfrog shows on its Web site, http://www.leapfroggroup.org, what hospitals voluntarily report to it in annual surveys. So far, most hospitals have chosen to report very little. I looked up the eight hospitals in our nation's capital where I live. Only one of the eight, Children's National Medical Center, responded to the 2008 survey. The others are all listed as "declined to respond" for Leapfrog's safety measures.[4]

If you live in an area with more forthcoming hospitals—Leapfrog says it has made most progress in populous states like California and Michigan—a wealth of data can be found in the Leapfrog hospital reports. But you have to drill down into the Web site to find it. On the main comparison page that lists all the hospitals in your area, you will find each safety item rated with a set of four green vertical bars, stepped up like the signal strength ratings you see on a cell phone. A hospital gets one short green bar just for being "willing to report," two bars for making "some progress," three for "substantial progress," and four for "fully meets standards." What's more interesting—at least to a fact junkie like me—is what you can see behind the individual ratings. Some of the categories have a very subtle *i* in a circle next to each hospital's cell-phone score; when you click on the *i* under the column "steps to avoid harm," you can see the hospital's actual score for compliance on each of the thirteen surveyed items. For example, you can find out if the hospital complies with the CDC handwashing guidelines (see Chapter 13), or the checklist of procedures to prevent catheter-related infections pioneered by Dr. Peter Pronovost (see page 179). And Leapfrog promises to make public at some point each hospital's rates of pressure ulcers and other preventable injuries—that is, for any hospitals willing to cough up the numbers voluntarily. Medicare, for its part, has those numbers but isn't publicizing them. Instead, Medicare in 2008 stopped paying hospitals for treatment of injuries that Medicare says are reasonably preventable: falls, pressure ulcers, and blood clots, to name a few. That might put pressure on hospitals to work harder to prevent these injuries, but in the meantime, it doesn't help us pick the safest, best hospitals.

The database should improve dramatically over the next decade, because a number of states have started mandating the reporting of injuries from "never events." Minnesota was the pioneer, in 2003. The list now includes California, Connecticut, Illinois, Indiana, New Jersey, Oregon, Washington, and Wyoming, according to the National Quality Forum, with more under consideration in state legislatures.

A Caveat About Big Brand-Name Hospitals

Another approach to finding the right hospital is to find the nearest brand-name institution. If you're in Minnesota or north Florida, that means the Mayo Clinic. The mid-Atlantic area: Johns Hopkins Hospital. And so on around the country. I wish it were that easy. Big, prestigious hospitals like M.D. Anderson in Houston (where Susan Scoble won a reprieve from her cancer death sentence) or Johns Hopkins in Baltimore, which I've mentioned favorably a couple of times, are not necessarily an easy shortcut to top-quality care. None of these hospitals is perfect; no institution of human beings can be. I've sued Hopkins on behalf of injured patients several times. In one, the care by a pediatric cardiologist was so bad, and so clearly caused the death of my clients' adorable three-year-old, that the hospital ran up the white flag shortly after we filed suit, and we reached a confidential settlement. You would make a mistake going to Hopkins without checking out the specific department and the specific doctor whose specialty covers what you need. The same applies wherever you live. The nearest mega-hospital connected to a medical school may or may not be right for you. Still, it's the place where I would start in looking for treatment for any serious disease, whether or not you may need surgery, because the mega–teaching hospital is most likely to have these critical ingredients for avoiding medical catastrophe and getting the best care:

- subspecialists in your disease and your kind of treatment,
- a research focus that helps assure up-to-date treatment,
- teams organized around these subspecialists to deliver the most coordinated care, and
- an institutional focus on preventing errors or catching them before they do harm.

But if you don't have an exotic condition and instead are laboring with garden-variety heart failure or diabetes or any of the other common ailments that fill hospitals, you may be better off with a good community hospital. How do we find the best?

A Radical Approach: Ask the Patients

This takes us to maybe the most radical but down-to-earth way to pick the best hospitals: Ask the patients what they think! I call this radical because it's brand-new. In its twenty years of rating hospitals, *U.S. News* has never asked a single patient what they think; its ratings of a hospital's reputation in a particular specialty is based mainly on what doctors in that specialty believe. But now Medicare has started requiring hospitals to have patients fill out a standardized survey when they leave the hospital, and the questions focus on a lot of issues that people care about and have a big impact on the quality and safety of their care:

- Did the doctors and nurses always communicate well?
- Was the bathroom always clean?
- Was your pain always well controlled?
- Was the area around your room always quiet at night?

Note that little word *always.* These are things patients have a right to expect—always.

To see how this works out in one real-life example, let's go to New Haven, Connecticut, home of Yale University. No, we're not going to Yale–New Haven Hospital, one of the nation's most prestigious medical institutions. Instead we'll drive due west ten miles to the Naugatuck River Valley town of Derby, where we find a hospital named Griffin.

Griffin Hospital gets great patient satisfaction ratings. *Fortune* magazine rated it one of the one hundred best places to work in America. And when you see a little of the hospital, you know why. Here's how Jim Conway, a top official with the Institute for Healthcare Improvement in Boston, one of the leaders in the field, enthuses about Griffin:

"Driving by, you wouldn't even notice it, very nondescript," says Conway. "But when you walk in the door you know you're in an extraordinarily different place. You'll see musicians playing in the lobby, a fireplace in the cafeteria, just a warm, welcoming environment. You go up to the unit, and you can not only look in your own chart whenever you want, you can write questions in the chart that you want the doctor or nurse to answer. It's also set up so families can choose whatever level of involvement they're comfortable with."

I found a lot of other impressive information about Griffin on its Web site, http://www.griffinhealth.org. A whole section on "performance indicators" includes all the publicly available numbers from Medicare, but also a lot of other numbers you don't often see hospitals publish. Griffin reports its infection rates associated with various types of surgery, ventilators, urinary catheters, and "central lines"; (tubes put into a major vein leading to the heart); it uses the central line practices pioneered by Dr. Peter Pronovost. Griffin's rate of 0 percent confirms Pronovost's research that these infections, which can be deadly, also can almost always be prevented.

The patient experience at Griffin includes daily delights such as visits from trained therapy dogs (from toy poodle to labs and golden retrievers), cookies and muffins baked by volunteers in kitchens on the patient units, strolling artists and musicians, back rubs, e-mail access for patients, a healing garden—the list goes on. It's almost enough to make you want to get sick in Connecticut so you can check in!

Griffin Hospital was completely remodeled in the early 1990s to incorporate the philosophy of a consumer health organization called Planetree, which takes its name from the tree under which Hippocrates sat teaching medical students in ancient Greece. Planetree is dedicated to humanizing health care by making it "patient-centered." Planetree has affiliated hospitals in thirty-one states; you can see a list at http://www.planetree.org. Griffin Hospital is Planetree's model of what an entire hospital thought out on patient-centered principles would look like.

To put the patient, rather than the doctor, at the center of the health-care experience, Planetree and Griffin did things like replace the traditional nurse's station on each unit, off limits to patients, with an open workplace that patients and families can use in addition to caregivers. The patient units are designed so that the patient's primary nurse is just outside the patient's door. Other aspects of the hospital are designed to cut the risk of patient falls, hospital infections, and medication errors, three of the biggest sources of preventable hospital injuries.

Griffin's ratings on the technical "process" indicators that we talked about earlier in this chapter are competitive with prestigious hospitals like Yale–New Haven. Where Griffin leaves the "top" hospitals in the dust, though, is the surveys of patient experiences, not just the warm fuzzy stuff—the therapy dogs and the cookies—but the key elements of a good hospital experience: communication and responsiveness. I looked up Griffin's patient survey ratings and compared them to Yale–New Haven and Johns Hopkins. (These survey numbers all can be found on the same Medicare Web site, http://www.hospitalcompare.hhs.gov, as the other technical data.) Johns Hopkins consistently scored a little better than Yale. This is what you'd expect for the number-one *U.S. News* hospital compared to number nineteen. But the real news was that unranked Griffin blew away both Yale and Hopkins in patient satisfaction in specific areas like communicating clearly, explaining medications, controlling pain, responding to the call button, and informing patients what to do at home.[5] These are the ABC's of high-quality, safe care that are so often overlooked in our doctor-centered, paternalistic health-care institutions.

Time for some caveats. Griffin is tiny, with 160 beds to Yale's 944 and Hopkins's 852 beds. Yale and Hopkins have huge arrays of super-specialist doctors—literally thousands of medical-school faculty members are on both hospitals' full-time staffs—and they offer a plethora of specialized services that Griffin cannot touch. But for everyday illnesses, including serious illnesses, Griffin shows that a consistent patient-centered philosophy can deliver safe, high-quality care.

If You Don't Live Near Griffin . . .

So what do I say to readers who don't live within driving distance of Griffin Hospital? You have to do your own research, using the tools discussed in this chapter and elsewhere in this book. Here's a plan of action for finding a hospital from the various aspects of safe, quality care that we've discussed.

1. Focus on how rare or common your condition is that you need the hospital for. The more unusual, the more you'll want to steer toward the top-reputation hospital in your area that has experience with your problem. There is no sense going to a hospital or doctor where you are going to be part of their learning curve. It can also make sense to do a regional or national search if there is no center of excellence for your condition in your immediate area.
2. For the great majority of conditions, you should be able to find safe, quality care in your own community. You still want to pay attention to volume if you need surgery; for major types of surgery, you can find numbers at http://www.hospitalcompare.hhs.gov.
3. Once you've satisfied yourself that your possible choices do enough of the kind of care you need, then next check the patient satisfaction surveys, also on hospitalcompare.hhs.gov; you have to go to the bottom of the report to find the patient survey. Focus mostly on the specific questions about the quality of communications and responsiveness to needs.
4. Look for a hospital affiliated with http://www.planetree.org, but if you find one, don't stop until you make sure it does okay on the next items on our checklist.
5. Next, look for specific "process" indicators that apply to your care. Two injury-prevention strategies that apply to almost every hospital patient are infection prevention and blood clot

prevention. The Medicare site, http://www.hospitalcompare.hhs.gov, has information for preventive antibiotics and blood clot strategies for surgery patients.

6. Check http://www.leapfroggroup.org for important quality indicators: computerized medication entry systems and full-time intensivists on staff in the ICU. Even if you don't go into an ICU, this quality measure was found in a study by Dr. Ashish Jha at Harvard to have a positive impact on overall quality as measured by lower death rates.
7. Look for the hospital's compliance with thirty "safe practices" from the National Quality Forum. You can find some information about this at http://www.leapfroggroup.org and more at the Joint Commission Web site.
8. You can also download a free accreditation report on any hospital from the Joint Commission, the main body that accredits hospitals in the United States at http://www.qualitycheck.org. Most of the data is a repeat of the Medicare "process quality" data, but you will also see how the hospital measures up on the set of thirty safe practices from the National Quality Forum. The Joint Commission's version of the Medicare data is a little more user-friendly than at Medicare's own Hospital Compare Web site; the Joint Commission report gives a comparison for how that hospital ranks both nationally and in its state on the "process" measures for heart attack care, heart failure care, and pneumonia care.
9. Some states are starting to require hospitals to publicly report their injury and infection rates. So you should check your own state's Web site for that information.

This plan is way more work than it should be. But that's what you have to do to save your own life as long as we have our current broken care system.

What about the thousands of same-day surgery centers that operate on millions of Americans every year? Unless they are hooked into a hospital's reporting system, you have little chance of finding out from public sources any useful information about them, other than the basics of whether they are accredited and licensed. You can and should ask the surgery center a series of questions focusing on safe surgery practices (see Chapter 11).

American health care has a long, long way to travel before patients will have enough information to let us make truly intelligent choices. Voluntary reporting by health-care institutions, especially when no one is auditing what they put out, just won't cut it. We need a uniform, mandatory public reporting system that generates for each hospital, clinic, and surgery center a report card of preventable injuries and deaths, patient satisfaction, and quality of care measures. Until we have that, at least you have some tools, and you know what to look for and what to ask.

Lifesavers:

Step Eight—Finding the Right Hospital

Finding the right hospital depends on what you are looking for. For exotic, unusual conditions, seek out the institution that has a lot of experience, and that may take you far from home. For common conditions—hip replacement, for example—you are much more likely to find the right fit near home. But you still have to make the match: volume of patients just like you, a dedicated team, a focus on key quality measures like infection control and ICU staffing, and maybe most important, the satisfaction of patients who came before you. Use the nine-part list on pages 199–200 for a comprehensive search strategy.

15

Living with Chronic Disease: Advice from Survivors

We have now reached Step Nine of our Necessary Nine steps for better medical care: *If you develop a chronic disease, educate yourself in what you need and learn how to audit your care to make sure you get it.* If you or a family member has a serious chronic illness, you already know that you must actively work your own health care. The stories that follow may help those who still live in the lucky land of full health to realize what they must do when that inevitable bridge looms ahead. I say inevitable because odds are that all of us, except for the immortal ones (ah, joyous fantasy!), will develop a serious long-term ailment of some kind. Those who have trod the path before you have important things to teach about learning to live with a terrible disease and all its aspects, both profound and mundane. We will also take one

> *Step Nine:*
> **If you develop a chronic disease, educate yourself in what you need and learn how to audit your care to make sure you get it.**

more hard look at medical statistics; I will show you how to find realistic hope in the numbers even when you have received the worst possible news.

Chad Roberts's Story

Chad Roberts's journey from life to fatal disease and back to life began when he nicked his skin shaving one morning just before Christmas. As the rivulet of blood continued to trickle down his neck, annoyance gave way gradually to alarm. It just would not stop. Finally at two o'clock in the afternoon, he called a doctor colleague at the law firm where he worked in Jacksonville, Florida. Dr. Sol Weinstein wrote a lab slip for Chad to have blood drawn for some standard blood counts and also some more exotic clotting factor tests. A day later, Chad stared at the sheet of results from the laboratory. At first he thought the paper had been misaligned in the printer, because all the numbers lined up below the "abnormal" heading at the top of the page. He had alarmingly low numbers of red cells, white cells, and particularly, nearly no platelets at all (which was why he couldn't clot his blood). He needed immediate medical treatment. *By the way*, he was told, *don't bump your head on the way to the hospital, because you could bleed to death with the slightest injury.*

As he took the first hesitant steps down the road of living with chronic disease, Chad Roberts had a choice. He could let his body drift, pushed here and there by the impersonal health-care system. Or he could get active. With a healthy push from his doctor colleague, he chose the active route. It started with the first phone call after the lab report was faxed to Chad. His regular doctors were fine, but Chad knew he needed to reach for the top. So his doctor friend called the hematology-oncology clinic at the Mayo Clinic in Jacksonville, the top-reputation facility in north Florida. It was almost funny, Chad recalls, as his doctor friend demanded "whoever's in charge there" come to the phone, but his bluster did win Chad a ticket to see one of the top doctors that same day.

The first discussions with the doctors, Chad recalls, "felt like an out-of-body experience. I was like floating, watching myself and watching the doctors talk about all these terrible things, and I wanted it to be someone else they were talking to, not me." But it wasn't someone else. Chad learned he had a type of leukemia, a cancer of the blood and bone marrow, called acute promyelocytic leukemia. Of the four types he could have, it was the most survivable, but only with four intense rounds of chemical bombardment of his blood-production system in his bone marrow. Each time, he was told, they would take his blood cells down to nearly nothing, and they would prop up his body with transfusions.

Because his white blood cells, the body's defender against infection, would be wiped out, the slightest infection could kill him. So Chad was told he could live in a hermetically sealed room at the hospital, with special ventilation so that the air always flowed outward, or he could create his own "bubble boy" environment at home. Home would actually be safer because of the nasty germs lurking in the hospital. So he chose home, and spent the next six months holed up in his bedroom, learning to touch no surfaces that had been touched by someone else, to eat no raw food or even be around any living plants (because even a wisp of fungus inhaled could rage through his body), and to wear a surgical mask every time he ventured out of the room. His closest companion was a digital thermometer; he had to take his own temperature every six hours, and did it twice with different thermometers to be double sure of the result. As soon as the temperature went up, he was under orders to bring himself to the emergency room because he would need heavy-duty intravenous antibiotics. In three of the four rounds of chemo, he did develop an infection, one of them a terribly serious sepsis in his bloodstream.

Just like Tony Benedi, whom we met in Chapter 2, Chad learned the key ingredient was to be inquisitive and ask a lot of questions. "They didn't mind it," he says. "The doctors and nurses actually kind of enjoyed explaining things. It just wasn't in their culture to explain unless you asked." It comforted him to know he had found some of the very best caregivers in his part of the country: "I received exemplary care from my treaters at Mayo Clinic. They were extremely bright young men and women very dedicated to the healing arts. Being there made a big difference." But that didn't stop him from asking questions, because he knew his treaters were just as human as everyone else.

Every time someone wanted to put something in his body, by injection or mouth, Chad ran through a mental checklist. Okay, is this medication for Chad Roberts? What is it? Are you sure I'm supposed to get it today? In this amount?

Chad also learned to actively manage the progress of his care. Once he knew what the landmarks or "set points" were—when the neutrophil level reaches 1,000, we will give you the next chemo drug—he found out that precious days would be wasted as his lab result would sit in his doctor's in-box. After a lot of pestering from Chad, they learned to call him with the results. Faster, better transitions from drug to drug came about.

Taking an active part in his care came naturally to Chad. He was forty-nine years old when his leukemia was found, a serious, studious, bespectacled lawyer who enjoyed working the little guy's side of David versus Goliath cases, a former engineer who had served on guided missile cruisers, which introduced him to the same kind of safety controls that we have discussed already in the aviation industry and that we have adapted for our nine-step approach to patient safety. In the Navy, safety is called the "two-intellect" approach, which means that any critical task has to involve two intellects, two humans, to double-check each other's work. "It's amazing," says Chad, "how advanced medicine is with its technology, but how far behind they are with the culture of safety. The Navy, on the other hand, has a culture of planning for mistakes. They know that every accident has eight links, say, leading up to it, and all you have to do is intervene at one of those links serendipitously and you can prevent the accident. So they would develop an intervention for each of those links."

As we have seen with other patients' stories in this book, like Sharon Burke and Lyn Gross and Helen F., tragedies almost never come out of a single error but from a cascade of mistakes by multiple caregivers. And one way to prevent injury, as we have discussed throughout, is for the patient to become actively involved with checking off the items of care that need to be done. That fits right in with the Navy's "two-intellect" approach.

Being an involved patient, Chad Roberts recognized, is just one of the interventions that can prevent an error. And Chad says, "I never got any real resistance. It never bugged them that I was so involved. It just wasn't part of their culture."

Chad Roberts emerged from his bubble after four successful but harrowing rounds of chemo, in July 2008. "I certainly don't want to take all the credit," he says now. "It's not like they were trying to kill me or anything. They have an excellent system, first-rate care, and I'm just glad that I could make it work better for me."

Louise Eisenbrandt's Journey of Discovery

Louise Eisenbrandt's first glimmer that something was wrong came one day when her hand holding a telephone shook so much she switched the phone to the other hand. She was fifty-seven years old. She had seen horror in emergency rooms in Vietnam as an army nurse tending soldiers. Now she lives with her husband, Jim, in a pleasant, leafy suburb of Kansas City called Overland Park, Kansas. She gardens, cooks, and enjoys photography—exactly the kind of lifestyle that you don't want to interrupt for a round of trips to doctors' offices looking for an answer to something that you tell yourself may be nothing. So Lou procrastinated for a few weeks and finally went to a neurologist recommended by her internist. His exam seemed thorough but he spent more time talking about his vacation than watching her tremor, and when three weeks went by with no report from the MRI scan, she called his office. Then she received an unproofed letter, filled with typos, that assured her that she did not have Parkinson's or dementia or a stroke, just some sort of nonspecific tremor. In other words, no diagnosis at all. She tried two drugs the neurologist recommended. One made her sleepy and didn't help; the other made her dizzy and also didn't help. Finally, at the urging of friends, and nagged by her doubts about the first neurologist, she sought another neurologist. Lou picks up the story:

"From the minute we met in her office, I could feel her gaze observing every movement, gesture, facial expression. She asked and listened. Then she said, 'I have good news and bad news. The bad news is that you have Parkinson's disease; the good news is that, since I began practicing in the 1960s, there have been many new medications to help control the symptoms.' I was astounded to learn that PD was not an 'old person's disease'; the average onset is fifty-five to sixty. I was fifty-seven. We addressed what the future held, which did *not* include medication at that early stage. I would soon learn that, because PD is progressive, it is important to not take more medication than needed in the early stages. As time passes, higher doses are required to control tremor or prevent stiffness. With those increased doses come greater side effects. A conservative approach to medication is the best approach—at least in my case. At the conclusion of that first visit, she gave me two pieces of advice. The first was, 'Exercise, exercise, exercise.' As a fitness enthusiast, that was the easy part. The second was, 'Rest every afternoon.' That was a much greater challenge and continues to be. However, this would be my life from here on and I vowed to do whatever it took to meet this new challenge."

Lou's journey with Parkinson's took its next turn the following Christmas after the diagnosis. That autumn had been stressful: a hospitalization for an unrelated blood clot in her leg, and her mother's death from metastatic breast cancer. Then when she was preparing Christmas dinner for close friends, she dropped a glass and it shattered. Her composure shattered with it. She started crying and could not stop. She called her neurologist the next day, who calmly said, "I think you need a little something for depression." Lou reflects, "With a background in nursing, I knew she was right." She continues, "The next few months were not my best. I had read much about the chemical depression that often accompanies PD. At the root of PD is the loss of dopamine—a substance in our brain that allows our body to run smoothly. I liken it to the oil in your car's engine; without it the vehicle will run, but only in fits and jerks. One of dopamine's main functions is to keep the body happy. With 80 percent of mine depleted, my body was anything but happy. The gray weather and cold temperatures of winter only added to my distress. As I adjusted to the antidepressant [citalopram], it was an effort just to get through the day."

Then she found a beacon of hope. It was called Turning Point,[1] a not-for-profit center in Kansas City that began in 2001 as a place for cancer patients to come together for classes on yoga, meditation, nutrition, and the other nonmedical but very important aspects of chronic illness. It quickly expanded to cover all serious ailments and to embrace family members and friends who needed support dealing with a loved one with a bad disease. Louise took classes there and attended support groups.

Lou says, "Surrounding myself with others who are in various stages of healing and coping is extremely helpful to my overall well-being. Whether it is listening to chemo recipients chuckling about their bald driver's license photos or writing comedic poetry about searching for lost libido, I am quickly realizing that laughter is indeed the best medicine. The center is filled with only optimism and enthusiasm."

Still, she faces challenges. There are the inevitable hassles with the insurance company, convincing it to cover a medicine she needs. She also wants to keep all her doctors informed when one of them changes a medication or does some other adjustment in treatment. Besides her neurologist, she has an allergist, an ear-nose-throat doctor, and a gynecologist. She sends identical faxes to each of them so they all know what the other is doing. This is her own form of centralized medical record (see Chapter 2).

Every day, Lou walks a treadmill two miles, lifts free weights, meditates, and does *jin shin jyutsu*, which she describes as acupuncture without the needles. She plays golf twice a week and sips the occasional glass of red wine. Every month, she gets a massage. She's done yoga, *tai chai*, and acupuncture. She joined the board of Turning Point, helping it raise money for its free courses and spreading the word about its resources, so she has now, as she puts it, "not just a resource for myself, but a new passion in my life and a cause to support."

Lou Eisenbrandt's final thoughts: "My prescription for facing health challenges is to be your own activist. Listen to your body's signals and to recommendations from people you trust. Then, ask questions and seek answers. Get a second or third opinion. Find physicians that you trust. Do they listen, ask questions, look you in the eye, return your calls, let you cry, share your laughter? When you are in their office, do you feel as though you have their undivided attention or are they standing by the door before you've finished sharing your latest ache or twitch? Surround yourself with friends who will support your decisions. Never take no for an answer. Remember: Life is short; do that which makes you happy!"

Patients Like You

You may have noticed something different about Chad's and Lou's stories. Chad focused on the technical aspects of his treatment: the blood levels of neutrophils, the next steps in the chemo—concrete, specific stuff. He is, after all, an engineer. Lou, the nurse who has tended the battle wounded, is much more in touch with the feelings in her mind and body: the emotional side. The group she's involved with, Turning Point, also is in tune with emotional support.

So when I tell you that a Web site called PatientsLikeMe (http://www.patientslikeme.com) was started by three MIT engineers, you already know it's filled with graphs, charts, and other bells and whistles. PatientsLikeMe began with a terrible disease called ALS, often referred to by the baseball star who became its namesake, Lou Gehrig. In 1998, when a twenty-nine-year-old carpenter named Stephen Heywood was diagnosed with ALS, his family began searching for treatments to extend his life and reduce the ravages of this mysterious disease that attacks nerves and gradually paralyzes the entire body. Victims lose the ability to walk, then to talk, then to move at all, and finally can communicate only by blinking their eyes in code.

The Heywoods and their friends put together the Web site to share treatment results. They have now expanded to include other neuromuscular diseases: Parkinson's and multiple sclerosis, plus HIV and mood disorders. Their mission is nothing less than this, to quote their Web site: "To create a community of patients, doctors, and organizations that inspires, informs, and empowers individuals. We're committed to providing patients with access to the tools, information, and experiences that they need to take control of their disease."[2]

When Todd Small, an MS victim from Seattle, clicked onto PatientsLikeMe, he discovered that there were two hundred other MS patients like him who took the muscle relaxant baclofen to cope with the muscle stiffness that made him feel sometimes like he was walking in quicksand.[3] More important, he found that his dose of ten milligrams was at the low end of the range of doses that others were taking, and this emboldened him to ask his neurologist to increase the dose, which his doctor had always told him needed to be kept as low as possible because it could weaken his muscles. They took the dose up to forty milligrams, and the quicksand episodes soon became more manageable.

That is what PatientsLikeMe offers that many other health-related Web sites, filled with advice from doctors and commiserating stories from fellow victims, don't have: hard data from individual patients on exactly what is happening with their medicines, dosages, and symptoms.

The approach is not for everyone. After an article in the *New York Times Magazine* in 2008, one reader wrote in that although she actively managed her own MS, she considered the Web site "a hypochondriac's virtual theme park"—overly obsessed with the day-to-day minutiae of symptoms. But to many other patients, PatientsLikeMe offers tools to help people become more than mere "patients," with all the passivity that word implies. People who join this Web site become comanagers of their disease treatment. And that can be a radical step forward. Or backward, in the wrong case. Notice I said "comanagers," not "managers." If becoming active in understanding and managing your disease makes you think you don't need your doctor's advice, because after all, what does he really know, then you need treatment for swollen-head syndrome, or a new doctor, or both. You can become an expert in your own body, but that doesn't give you the objectivity and knowledge to always know what's best for you. It's like the lawyer who represents himself and has a fool for a client. It's better to team up with a comanager rather than try to run the show all by yourself. (See Chapter 5 on finding a top primary-care doctor for more on this.)

One other feature of PatientsLikeMe deserves underscoring, because it fits with something I've tried to do with this book: Tell you stories about real people using their real names. Privacy is a good thing, but too much privacy in the medical setting can harm us by making it harder to share knowledge and by making us feel embarrassed and ashamed. The writer Susan Sontag put her finger on this when she published *Illness as Metaphor*[4] about her experience with breast cancer. She wrote, "Any disease that is treated as a mystery and acutely enough feared will be felt to be morally, if not literally, contagious. Contact with someone afflicted with a disease regarded as a mysterious malevolency inevitably feels like a trespass; worse, like the violation of a taboo." She said she wanted to cure this stigma by "demythicizing" the disease. That, in a sense, is a large part of my mission with this book. Once you start down the path of active involvement in your health care with Step One of our Necessary Nine steps, by getting and reading your medical records, you have started breaking down the barriers of shame and taboo that still lurk around disease and around people who become sick.

The PatientsLikeMe folks put the idea this way: "We believe sharing your healthcare experiences and outcomes is good. Why? Because when patients share real-world data, collaboration on a global scale becomes possible. New treatments become possible. Most importantly, change becomes possible. At PatientsLikeMe, we are passionate about bringing people together for a greater purpose: speeding up the pace of research and fixing a broken healthcare system. Currently, most healthcare data is inaccessible due to privacy regulations or proprietary tactics. As a result, research is slowed, and the development of breakthrough treatments takes decades. Patients also can't get the information they need to make important treatment decisions. But it doesn't have to be that way. When you and thousands like you share your data, you open up the healthcare system. You learn what's working for others. You improve your dialogue with your doctors. Best of all, you help bring better treatments to market in record time."

Outliving Your Life Expectancy

An ambitious agenda, to be sure. But you don't necessarily have to buy into PatientsLikeMe's grand, world-rattling vision to realize that this approach can help at least one person who matters most: you, or one of your loved ones. That happened to my neighbor Lila Snow. When her husband, George, a high-energy particles physicist and a professor at the University of Maryland, came down with a fatal blood cancer called myeloid metaplasia, Lila's involvement with his care helped him live another ten years. The usual patient can succumb to this disease in two or three years. Lila is a white-haired artist, a builder of collages, who in her youth worked as a medical technician. Decades later, when the diagnosis came in, Lila went to a stationery store and bought a diary. She filled its blank pages with neat tables of George's blood counts from his lab, and she made graphs to show the ups and downs of his white count. When the cancer doctor, a superior, brusque type who was always in a hurry, proclaimed that there was no need for medication because the white count was doing fine, she was ready to show him the data that proved the white count was skyrocketing. Lila, a strong-willed, independent soul, soon found this doctor so off-putting that she stopped going to the appointments with her husband. But she did two things that were important: She prepared her husband for each visit with all the latest numbers from his tests, and she also sent him to get a second opinion from a leading expert in this type of cancer. The reason she bird-dogged the lab results so closely, Lila says, is simple: "I only had one patient. But George's doctor had too many to keep track of some details."

Beating the Numbers Starts with Understanding Them

George Snow outlived his life expectancy thanks to his wife Lila's focus on him as her sole patient. Earlier in this book, we saw how cancer patients like Susan Scoble and Elmer Wischmeier proved the predictions of their imminent demise were wrong. Cancer is slowly becoming a chronic disease like a lot of others, that people can live with for a long time.

When you read about how far off the doctors' estimates of life expectancy have been, you could be forgiven for thinking that the doctors who pronounced the premature death sentences must have been idiots. But that's not the real problem. A closer look at medical statistics shows why these stories are so common, and what you need to look for in the numbers if you or a loved one has just received bad medical news. We have visited medical statistics in Chapter 7, about how the numbers behind "breakthrough" drugs can be so misleading, and in Chapter 8, on what you need to know about "false positives" and "false negatives" in medical testing. Now, I want to show you one more lesson on how to understand the reality of medical statistics by, as we have done before, "counting the people."

When a patient with a terrible diagnosis asks a doctor, "How long do I have?" the doctor's response is usually to quote averages. A precise answer would be something like, "The median survival time for people who have the disease at your stage is eight months" (or whatever the number is). Too many stunned patients translate that into "I have eight months to live at most." That's a mistake—but it can turn into a self-fulfilling prophecy if you give up before you understand what the number means. *Median* refers to the halfway mark in a group of people. If patient A lives one month, patient B two months, patient C eight months, patient D twenty-four months, and patient E thirty-six months, the median survival time in that group of five is eight months—the point where half lived shorter and half lived longer. This hypothetical group of patients is not far off from the wide range that researchers find when they put together survival data for large numbers of patients—it varies a lot from short to long. Some simple lessons:

- Statistics are just compilations of individual experiences. But everyone is different. The median is just a convenient way to measure average-ness; it's not a pronouncement of where you are going to end up.
- Another way to measure average is the *mean*. In our group of five patients, the mean survival is 14.2 months (1 + 2 + 8 + 24 + 36 divided by the number of patients, 5, equals 14.2). But nobody lived that long; again, everyone is different.
- Notice that neither measure of average—median or mean—tells you what you really want to know: What are my realistic prospects for beating the average? In our group of five, 40 percent (two of the five) lived at least twenty-four months. Somebody who realizes he has a good shot at living two years is a lot better situated emotionally than someone who thinks he has a maximum of eight months.

Key Questions to Ask about Survival Numbers

The bottom line for proactive patients is to never settle for average, and never settle for a simple number, because one size never fits all. You need to count the people. Here's what you want to know:

- How many patients were in the group that the statistics came from? (The smaller the numbers, the more likely they could be misleadingly grim. I used a hypothetical group of five just to teach some basics. You want to see compilations on the order of thousands of patients if possible.)

- How like or different were these people from me?
- What was the range of experience? How many lived one year, two years, three years, more?

What you really want to know is, how do I get into that group of longer-lived patients? That takes the kind of research that we described in Chapters 5 and 10 to find the right doctor with the right treatment, and the strategy we'll develop in the next chapter about devising an audit for your key care needs.

The Median Is Not the Message

Stephen Jay Gould, the famous Harvard evolutionary biologist, found out that he had a rare cancer and that median survival was eight months. He lived another twenty years, and died from an unrelated cause. Gould wrote an elegant essay about how he explored the statistics of his disease. He called it, with apologies to Marshall McLuhan, "The Median Isn't the Message." You can find it, and other excellent advice about how to do your own cancer research, on a great Web site, http://www.cancerguide.org, developed by a patient named Steve Dunn. Dunn came down with kidney cancer and was terrified to read that the odds of surviving one year were under 10 percent. He worked up his own death-defying strategies and lived fifteen more years, dying eventually from an unrelated cause. You can read these stories, and ones in this book, and conclude, as the nineteenth-century British prime minister Benjamin Disraeli did, that "there are three kinds of lies: lies, damned lies, and statistics." But that would be wrong. On his Web site, Dunn wrote that it might feel natural to just reject scary statistics outright, but they are useful as guides and motivators—particularly when you focus, as I urge, on the raw numbers of actual numbers of people who live for a particular amount of time. (Remember: Count the people.) Dunn's bottom line applies to all of us: "Statistics outline probabilities—they cannot limit possibilities."

Lifesavers:

Beating the Odds

To live successfully with a chronic disease, as we all someday must (personally or through a family member), we must learn some basic strategies. The first adapts Dylan Thomas's advice to his father: "Do not go gentle into that good night; rage, rage against the dying of the light." Not the anger part, perhaps, but the determination—the will to put ourselves out at the right end of the curve of survival by finding out what other survivors have done to stretch their odds toward the light. Will is followed by questions, and questions, pounded hard by thorough research, give way to answers. In our next chapter, we will look at further ways to implement a successful strategy for coping with chronic disease.

16

Auditing Your Care so You Live Longer

For any chronic disease, the best medical care is light-years better than the mediocre care inflicted on most people with that disease. You can use the general techniques from Chapter 4 for finding a primary-care doctor who specializes in your illness. But you can do a lot better for yourself by learning the basics of what the care for your condition should consist of and then do an audit to make sure you get it. For many of the most common diseases, finding the "right stuff" is simpler than you might think. If you have an aging parent with a chronic condition, read this chapter for the ways you can help them. Carrying through with this final Step Nine of our Necessary Nine will prepare you to extend the twilight years for your loved ones and yourself, and we all know that twilight can be a magical, special time.

A Story of Preventable Blindness from Diabetes

You would know in the first minute of meeting Genevieve Porter (I changed the name at her request) that she was not the type to ask probing questions of her internist. She was retired from working as a housekeeper at a government building, a quiet, polite, uncomplaining widow who lived alone in a trim two-story brick home. She volunteered at church and enjoyed tending her tomato patch in the summer. For thirteen years, she caught the bus every three months to the office of her internist, whom I will call Dr. Flint. He drew blood for a fasting blood sugar. At first he had her take oral diabetes medication but then switched to twice-daily insulin injections, which his nurse taught her. Every now and again he would call her a few days after the blood sugar report came back and tell her to adjust the mix of short-acting and long-acting insulins that she took. When she started to lose her eyesight, he told her it was a natural consequence of the diabetes, and she accepted that. It was only after her second, unsuccessful eye surgery that her son Tommy insisted she switch to a diabetes specialist. The new doctor was shocked that she had never heard of daily blood sugar home monitoring and surprised that she had never received annual eye examinations while her vision was still good.

My introduction to Dr. Flint came through his medical records for Mrs. Porter. He first saw her in October 1985, just after the internist across the hall in a strip-mall building had died. The widow had sold the practice to Dr. Flint, and Mrs. Porter stayed with Dr. Flint for the next thirteen years until she became legally blind. When I questioned Dr. Flint in a deposition, I was able to ask him detailed questions that few patients are persistent enough to ask. I learned that he considered himself a cardiologist, although he lacked board certification in cardiology or the parent board of internal medicine, that he had flunked the internal medicine board four times, and that he had finally given up the effort to become board certified. To keep his medical license, he had to take a few hours of continuing education each year, but could recall no specific diabetes refresher course, although he regularly saw hundreds of diabetes patients a year. He subscribed to no medical journals and claimed he kept up with new developments by going to the library once a year. He wasn't on the staff of any of the three hospitals near his office. In short, he worked alone, isolated from his colleagues, without any regular exposure to modern methods of diabetes care. Dr. Flint's approach, which he had learned at a medical school in the Caribbean, was to worry only if the patient had blood sugar so low or so high that it threatened immediate coma or death. He missed all the advances in diabetic care in the 1970s and 1980s when doctors learned that if they kept blood sugar tightly controlled with multiple daily testing and adjustment of insulin doses, they could greatly reduce the ravages that diabetes causes to the body's tiny blood vessels, and in turn, to the kidneys, eyes, nerves, and feet. Diabetes treaters also learned that regular visits to an ophthalmologist, with a dilated-pupil exam of the eyes, could lead to early detection of diabetic changes in the retina of the eye, and laser treatment to prevent blindness.

The diabetes statistics are stunning. The people with new, preventable consequences of diabetes could populate small cities every year: 24,000 new cases of adult-onset blindness, more than any other preventable disease-related blindness; 82,000 foot amputations; and many thousands of heart attacks, strokes, and kidney failures as a result of excess sugar in the blood choking off blood supply to important organs. Nearly all of these complications, espeically those caused by damage to small arteries, can be prevented or put off until deep in old age by tight sugar control and regular tests for early signs of complications.

Dr. Flint tried to blame Mrs. Porter, even though he also called her "one of my favorite patients, a very outgoing, effervescent person." He said she refused to do home blood sugar testing and to go on a special diabetic diet. He brushed off the wildly high results on his fasting blood sugar tests because he claimed she routinely would sip orange juice before he took the sample. He maintained that his records were silent about this alleged noncompliance because he hadn't wanted to write down anything negative about her. (When I told Mrs. Porter what he said, I watched her brow wrinkle in disbelief, and then she softly shook her head from side to side. "*Mm, mm, mm,*" was all she could say.) He had more trouble explaining why he had never taken a key test called hemoglobin A1C, which is far superior to the fasting blood-sugar test because it gives an indicator of the average amount of sugar in the blood for the past few weeks instead of the snapshot view that the fasting test gives of a single moment on a single day.

Genevieve Porter went slowly blind from diabetic retinopathy. Tiny blood vessels grow abnormally to feed the starved retina and actually lift off the retina from the back wall of the eye. It's a process that takes many years and is totally preventable, with both tight blood sugar control[1] and laser treatments[2] to seal off the abnormal small vessels when they start growing into the retina.

I showed Dr. Flint's tattered, disorganized, elliptical records to experts in diabetes care. They pronounced his practice appalling, inexcusable, but fairly typical of what many general practitioners inflict on their diabetic patients. The only way that patients can bring their blood sugar under good control is with home blood sugar testing and regular, sometimes daily phone calls with the doctor until they learn how to manage their bodies' sugar rhythms. Many general practitioners don't have the time or inclination for such close work with their patients, but they enjoy the steady income from the regular visits of diabetic patients, and so millions of diabetics receive indifferent care that will shorten and hobble their lives. You think I exaggerate? The two most comprehensive surveys of diabetes patients in the last ten years found that one in four patients in one study, and three in ten in the other, had had their hemoglobin A1C tested in the previous year. The number should be close to 100 percent, since this test has been a benchmark of quality diabetes care since the late eighties. [3]

The American Diabetes Association has done its part to try to educate practitioners on the components of high-quality care. Unlike many other medical societies, which try to shield their members from accountability by softening every recommendation into a "guideline" and by sprinkling legal disclaimers throughout these documents, the Diabetes Association minces no words. It identified the hemoglobin A1C test (also called glycosolated hemoglobin), at least twice a year, as a "standard of medical care" in 1989; it called for annual eye exams for all diabetics even earlier than that.

The goal is to bring the hemoglobin A1C under 7 percent; patients who can keep it there reduce their long-term risk of blindness by fourfold.[4] The annual eye tests are also critical because once you notice visual loss, it's too late. The time to attack the abnormal blood vessels is when they're at the periphery of the retina and haven't yet started to interfere with central vision.

If you've read this far in this chapter, you now know two of the top three indicators of quality diabetes care that were published in a landmark study that audited quality of care in thirty important diseases.[5] (The third of the three is that any diabetic who has protein in the urine, which means the kidneys aren't filtering correctly, should be treated with a high-blood-pressure drug from the family called "ACE inhibitors" or another family called ARB drugs, because that can halt the progression of loss of kidney function.) You can use these indicators to audit the quality of your own care. Let me tell you a little more about where these quality indicators come from and some specific practical examples of their use.

A Landmark Survey of Health-Care Quality

Researchers from the RAND Corporation, headed by Elizabeth McGlynn, asked panels of medical experts to list the top quality of care indicators for all the leading causes of death, disability, and doctor/hospital visits. They scoured the published research and came up with 439 indicators in thirty categories of disease. You can read all of the indicators, organized alphabetically by disease, by downloading the document from the RAND Web site.[6] This is a technical document, but it only takes a little bit of translation to make it workable for laypeople. Besides listing the top-quality indicators, it also rates them on a scale from one to three: one for the indicators most proven by gold-standard, randomized, controlled studies to make a big difference in health outcomes; two for nonrandomized controlled trials; three for the ones that have drawn a consensus of expert opinion and make a lot of sense but lack rigorous test data to back them up. This work by Dr. McGlynn and her team has proven the "half-nots" of American medical care that we discussed in Chapter 1 of this book. Since your odds of not getting all the care you need for your chronic disease are on the order of fifty-fifty ("half-not"), it pays to know more about what top experts think your kind of disease deserves by way of routine care.

Auditing Heart-Attack Care

Let's look at the most common killer of adult Americans: heart attack. Every sixty-five seconds, someone dies in the United States from a heart attack. It's responsible for one in five deaths. About 7.2 million men and 6 million women live with coronary-artery disease.[7] In these people, the arteries that course across the surface of the heart, feeding oxygen to the heart muscle, become narrowed over many years by plaque lining the inside of the arteries. When a plaque breaks open, a blood clot suddenly forms and blocks flow to the muscle downstream, killing that section of the heart. The greater the blockage, the bigger the damage. Doctors treat heart attack by a combination of treatments intended to reduce formation of blood clots, break up clots that have already formed, and help the heart recover by smoothing out the heart rate. That means the following at a minimum. This is the auditable list of top treatments, all proven by randomized studies to save lives and reduce heart damage:

- *Aspirin coming into the hospital and aspirin going home.* Aspirin is a lifesaver for the heart (and the brain, as we'll discuss later) because it blocks the stickiness of platelets, the particles that form the first layer of blood clots. If you think of a platelet as a piece of Velcro, aspirin knocks out one section of the Velcro, and Plavix, also an antiplatelet drug, knocks out another, so they're often used together for maximum antistickiness. But the absolute minimum standard, unless you're allergic to aspirin or have problems taking it, is to take an aspirin within two hours of arriving at the emergency room, and then receive instructions to continue taking it every day when you go home.[8]

- *A beta-blocker drug coming in and going out.* Beta-blockers smooth out the heart rhythm and slow the heartbeat and thus help protect the heart after a heart attack. This is another minimum standard unless there's a very good reason not to give it.[9]
- *Clot-busting drugs as soon as possible.* These drugs can chew up a clot that already exists, unlike aspirin, which just helps keep the clot from getting bigger. The problem is they do no good unless given within twelve hours of the onset of symptoms of a heart attack.[10]
- *ACE inhibitor drug on discharge if heart pumping is impaired.* Of the four chambers of the heart, the one whose pumping you will see measured most is the left ventricle, the workhorse that pushes freshly oxygenated blood into the aorta and from there to the entire body. The volume of blood ejected with each beat divided by the volume of blood in the ventricle just before the contraction is called the ejection fraction, and in a normal person is above 55 percent; that means that with each beat, the heart should pump 55 percent or more of the blood in the left ventricle out to the body. If it's under 40 percent at any time during a heart attack hospitalization, an ACE inhibitor drug should be prescribed at discharge.[11] These drugs help compensate for the reduced pumping efficiency of the heart by increasing the volume of blood ejected by each contraction and lowering the resistance of the tiny arteries in muscles, making it easier to feed blood to the body.

So, you have just absorbed a short course in heart attack and its proven treatments. If everyone who had a heart attack received these treatments in a reliable and consistent way, the only point in this lesson might be to show that sophisticated medical knowledge is not all that hard to come by. Which itself is a valuable point, inasmuch as so many people let themselves be intimidated by the medical system into surrendering their normal inquisitiveness. But the fact is that Americans do not receive these proven treatments with nearly the reliability that we deserve and should expect. Beta-blockers, for example, were used for fewer than half of the heart attack victims surveyed by the RAND study, although these drugs have been proven to cut the risk of death by 13 percent in the first week of treatment and by 23 percent over the long haul. Aspirin was offered to only six in ten patients, although it has been shown to reduce the risk of a repeat heart attack by 30 percent and the risk of a nonfatal stroke by 40 percent. (One of the downstream risks after a heart attack is stroke, because the weakened heart muscle can produce clots that shoot up to the brain and clog key arteries).[12]

A Diabetes-Care Audit

An educated public could go a long way toward boosting the numbers of patients who win these proven treatments. But one problem is that the easily auditable lists of effective treatments are not all that easy to come by. I checked out one popular Web site for diabetics: MyDiabetes Central.com (http://www.healthcentral.com/diabetes/), part of the www.healthcentral.com group of sites that publishes lay-oriented information from medical specialists and informed patients, and that lets readers write in questions and receive at least a sympathetic ear. I was looking for the place on the site that informed diabetics of the proven treatments that work to cut their risk of the devastating long-term complications of diabetes, like losing their kidneys, their vision, their feet. It turned out to be scattered in different places; the key advice about getting an annual eye exam, for example, appears on the last page of a long article called "long-term complications."[13] The same information about annual eye exams is easier to find on the American Diabetes Association site, but you still have to look for it. I found it in an article called "Who's on Your Health Care Team?" in a section about your first visit after the diabetes diagnosis.[14]

The RAND list strips away all the fluff and gets quickly to the key items of diabetes care: the three top-rated items we already discussed (hemoglobin A1C, annual eye exam, and ACE inhibitor blood pressure drugs for anyone with protein in the urine), plus nine others I've added in the endnote.[15]

So there's power and usefulness in the RAND list of proven treatments. You have to deal with some medical jargon to use the list, but at least you don't have to wander through multiple layers of complex Web sites, fending off pop-up ads and sundry Internet clutter, just to find the list. The information in the RAND list is easily found, is authoritative, and deserves wide use by proactive patients checking the markers for their own health-care quality. Another good source of authoritative guidance is the National Guideline Clearinghouse, at http://www.guidelines.gov, which compiles consensus reports on the best way to treat more than 2,000 diseases.

I'm not the only one who wants you to use these benchmark treatments to audit the quality of your health care. The federal government is another. As we discussed in Chapter 14, Medicare launched a Web site in 2005 that compares hospitals on some of the same quality items that the RAND researchers developed. Its Web site, http://www.hospitalcompare.hhs.gov, has "process" ratings for four common conditions: heart attack, heart failure (weakness of the pumping action of the heart), pneumonia, and prevention of surgical infections.

Lifesavers:

Getting Started with Your Own Health-Care-Quality Audit

Chad Roberts, Louise Eisenbrandt, the folks at PatientsLikeMe, and so many other pioneers teach us that when it comes to living with a chronic disease, knowledge is power. And another necessary predicate is this: You are not alone. The research is out there, on patients just like you, and it is not that hard to find. Once you find the knowledge, you can insist that you receive what you know you need.

Here are the thirty conditions (plus one more category for general preventive care) for which you can find objective auditing standards in the RAND Corporation study. I give first the medical jargon term used by RAND followed by a translation, if necessary, in parentheses:

alcohol dependence

asthma

atrial fibrillation (a chronic heart rhythm disturbance in the chamber called the atrium)

BPH (benign prostatic hypertrophy—non-cancerous enlargement of the prostate gland)

breast cancer

CAD (coronary artery disease—blockage of the arteries that feed the heart)

cancer pain and palliation

Cesarean delivery

CHF (congestive heart failure)

colorectal cancer

community-acquired pneumonia

COPD (chronic obstructive pulmonary disease)

CVD (cerebral vascular disease—stroke)
depression
diabetes
dyspepsia/PUD (peptic ulcer disease)
headache
hip fracture
hyperlipidemia (high cholesterol)
hypertension (high blood pressure)
hysterectomy
low-back pain
menopause management
orthopedic conditions
osteoarthritis
prenatal care
preventive care
prostate cancer
senile cataract (of the eye lens)
STDs/vaginitis (sexually transmitted diseases)
UTI (urinary tract infection)

You can pull the list of quality treatments for each of these thirty conditions from the RAND Web site.[16]

For further authoritative research guidance, I recommend http://guidelines.gov, an ongoing project of the U.S. Department of Health and Human Services, and http://www.uptodate.com, a private consortium of medical specialty organizations that regularly compiles the latest research on what works and what doesn't work. See Resources, pages 257–260 for more.

17

Celebrating the Heroes and Champions of Patient Safety and Quality Care

Our tour through the fragmented health-care system has taught us that patients need to take things into our own hands if we want to secure the best treatment for ourselves and our families. One day we will have a better, safer, more comprehensive health-care system that maintains high-quality standards, discloses mistakes openly, and makes no excuses for poor performance. We've traveled a few inches down the road, with many miles yet to go. This final chapter shines the spotlight on heroes and champions of health-care reform. The heroes are people who have seen terrible things happen to a family member and who have vowed to do whatever they can to make sure the same thing doesn't happen to someone else. They are by and large laypeople who have educated themselves in our health-care system. The champions are health-care professionals who are devoting their careers to finding innovative ways to bring American health care up to the uniform quality standards that Americans have a right to expect. Here are a few of the many whose work we can all take heart from.

Sorrel King: Mother, Hero, Pioneer of the Family-Activated Rapid-Response Team

Whenever I have represented a young couple who has lost a small child, I have marveled at how they can manage. When a child has died from the neglect of doctors or nurses who had pledged to help that child through an illness, the feeling of betrayal is overpowering. When Sorrel King's youngest child, Josie, died at age eighteen months, at one of the world's top medical institutions, Johns Hopkins Hospital in Baltimore, rage overwhelmed her. But then she turned her anger into something positive. Sorrel, a former fashion designer, and her husband Tony, a financial wiz, took some of the money that Hopkins paid in a settlement of their legal claim and started a patient-safety foundation.[1] The foundation has a laser focus on one specific change that would have saved Josie King's life. It's called a family-activated "rapid-response team."

The idea of a rapid-response team is one step down from the drama of a Code Blue team that comes running into a patient's room to pump life back into the patient after the heart has stopped. A rapid-response team is designed to head off the need to call a Code Blue by getting to the patient when the condition is deteriorating but a full-blown emergency hasn't yet happened. And the most important part of the innovation is that the patient's family can summon the rapid-response team any time they think things aren't going right. At the University of Pittsburgh Medical Center, which has worked with the Kings, they call it "Condition H—for Help." When a Condition H is declared, a doctor, nurse coordinator, patient-relations specialist, and a floor nurse all come to the bedside within minutes and address whatever crisis the family believes is occurring. You can read more about the Pittsburgh program on the Josie King Foundation Web site.[2] So many leaders have been impressed with the idea that the state of

Massachusetts now mandates rapid-response teams, and the Web site of the Leapfrog Group has a check-off box for each hospital on its survey to show whether or not the hospital has a rapid-response team. Sorrel King is convinced that Josie would still be alive if Hopkins had had a rapid response team. Sorrel saw her daughter sucking on a washrag and knew something was terribly wrong, but she couldn't get the attention of the busy staff until it was too late. It turned out the toddler had advanced dehydration.

The key lesson that Sorrel King is teaching to doctors all over the country: Listen to the family. They know when their child doesn't look right. And when families are empowered to call in a "rapid-response team," it will be a win-win: better care for the patient, better focus for distracted caregivers, and better peace of mind for the family.

Sue Sheridan: Mother, Wife, Hero—and Messenger of the Healing Power of Honesty

Sue Sheridan knows too well the insult piled on injury when doctors don't admit what they've done wrong and instead hide the truth. It happened twice to her, once when her son suffered preventable brain damage shortly after birth and the second when her husband's brain cancer was misdiagnosed because a pathology report was lost. Both times the feeling of loss and betrayal nearly tore her family apart. Her son survived, but with serious handicaps, and today lives with Sue in Eagle, Idaho, but her husband, Pat, died of his brain cancer. On his deathbed, Sue says, Pat Sheridan told her never to give up on patient safety, and Sue Sheridan responded by starting not one but two patient-advocacy groups. The first came out of her son's experience with a brain-poisoning jaundice a few days after birth; the disease is called kernicterus, and her group is called Parents of Infants and Children with Kernicterus (PICK), and can be found at http://www.pickonline.org. The second group is Consumers Advocating Patient Safety (CAPS), which Sue Sheridan co-founded with Martin Hatlie, a Chicago attorney who represented doctors and hospitals in malpractice cases.

CAPS, whose Web site is http://www.patientsafety.org, advocates for a number of reforms to end the secrecy of malpractice settlements and establish a national patient safety authority with power to monitor and enforce safety changes. I don't agree with all the reforms proposed by this group, which to me is a little too closely aligned with the medical establishment, but it does a good job of putting patient safety onto the public agenda.

Sue Sheridan's experience with her son Cal's birth in 1995 was especially tragic because his severe cerebral palsy, crossed eyes, hearing impairment, and inability to speak were all 100 percent preventable. Sue and her husband as new parents didn't know better that severe jaundice can be a medical emergency and can cause brain damage. Jaundice, which is the yellow color in the skin and the whites of the eyes, comes from bilirubin, a product of the liver that at excessive levels can invade brain tissue. Six in ten babies are born with jaundice, and most do fine with adjustments in their diet or a spell under the photo lamps (bright light on the skin detoxifies bilirubin). But if the baby becomes lethargic, develops a high-pitched cry, and arches the back, those are all signs that brain damage is starting to occur and aggressive treatment is needed, including exchange transfusion to take out all the bilirubin circulating in the baby's bloodstream. Cal Sheridan had skin nearly as dark as a pumpkin, and three days after birth, he started to show all the classic signs that brain damage was starting. But his parents didn't know, and the hospital and pediatricians treated it as routine jaundice. Worse, the parents were lied to about the results of a brain MRI, which they were told was normal. Eighteen months later, at wit's end because of their son's strange development and behaviors, they took Cal to an academic medical center. They collected his records to take to the doctors, and when they actually read the MRI report, it said he had classic signs of kernicterus brain damage.

(Every potential parent or grandparent needs to know about jaundice-related brain damage because it's so preventable. I recommend an excellent Web site written by a physician who has devoted his career to preventing kernicterus. His name is Steven Shapiro, MD, a pediatric neurologist at Virginia Commonwealth University in Richmond, and the site is http://www.kernicterus.org/.)

Sue Sheridan wrote movingly about the feelings that she and her husband felt after seeing the MRI report that finally gave them the truth about their son that had been hidden for eighteen months: "I can only describe it as a hit-and-run health-care accident. My family was abandoned at the side of the road, injured and traumatized by a well-meaning motorist who fled because of legal and personal fears. We were left to seek out help on our own with our own resources. No one looked back. They pretended as if nothing had happened. . . . A hit and run, in our world, is considered criminal. Why is it okay in medicine? The nondisclosure of medical error is the most destructive phenomenon in health care. Trust and confidence disappear in a heartbeat."[3]

The failure to disclose the truth to her family, Sue Sheridan said, made it hard to heal from the betrayal. "The calculated dishonesty to protect their money and pride is at the very core of the challenge I face to forgive. It is this forgiveness that we need to move on."

Her message, when she speaks to hospital administrators and trustees, is:

"Have the courage to be honest. Disclosure and transparency are simply a new kind of glitzy way to say the word *honesty*, and I know of no other industry where honesty is optional."

Cathy Lake: Daughter, Hero—and Firefighter

Kernicterus is one of the "never events" that the National Quality Forum says should never happen in America. Another "never event" is setting the patient on fire during surgery. This sounds so bizarre it's almost funny, but it happened to Cathy Lake's mother, and it happens to an estimated four patients every week in American hospitals.

Cathy's mom was Catherine Barahona Reuter, a native of El Salvador who came to the United States at age twenty, served as a Catholic nun for twenty-two years, teaching bilingual kindergarten and first grade in the San Francisco area, then left the sisterhood, got married and had two children. At age sixty-nine, she entered a major Washington, D.C., hospital for heart valve surgery. Cathy Lake remembers the surgeon telling her there had been a fire in the operating room. She assumed it was in some debris in a corner. No, the fire was on her mother's skin, and she had inhaled flames into her throat. How did this happen? They used a flammable alcohol-based skin prep to wash the skin and didn't wait until it evaporated before they started using an electro-cautery device, which ignited the fumes. Why use a flammable solution instead of old-fashioned, nonflammable Betadine? The alcohol-based solutions are favored in many operating rooms because they dry colorlessly, unlike Betadine, which leaves an orange cast on the skin that has to be scrubbed off.

Oxygen is another thing that can cause fires and explosions in operating rooms. Fires can happen when oxygen is used in too high a concentration near the electro-cautery device, which is used to seal bleeding blood vessels. Or the oxygen, which is an odorless and colorless gas, can leak and accumulate under drapes, ready to be touched off by a drill, a laser, or another trigger.

Thanks to Cathy Lake's drumbeat of publicity and prodding of medical organizations, the Joint Commission, which accredits hospitals, issued a "sentinel alert" about the risks of surgical fires, and the American Society of Anesthesiologists in 2008 issued a "practice advisory" about how to prevent OR fires. [4] You can read more on her Web site: http://www.surgicalfire.org.

Cathy Lake's lesson for all patients and families: If you find something that needs fixing, you can fix it. Don't be intimidated by not having a medical degree. This is the patients' health-care system, not just the doctors'.

Nancy Conrad: Wife, Hero—Communicator

Nancy's husband, Pete Conrad, commanded the second Apollo landing on the moon and flew three other missions into space. He was one of the main astronauts featured in Tom Wolfe's *The Right Stuff.*

"If you can't be good," he used to say, "be colorful." According to Nancy, he was both. In July 1999, Pete Conrad was involved in a motorcycle accident and suffered some broken ribs. Nancy took the phone call and went to the small rural hospital to wait to see him after he left the operating room. After what seemed like hours, a physician came out, asked, "Which of you is Mrs. Conrad?" and then said, "He's dead." And walked out. Later, much later, she learned that her husband had died from a series of oversights that delayed the treatment of bleeding inside his chest.

In her grief and anger, Nancy Conrad founded a group called Community Emergency Healthcare Initiative, to try to reduce needless deaths in emergency rooms. Her group gives Pete Conrad Patient Safety Excellence Awards every year to researchers and leaders in the patient safety movement. She gives talks advocating for openness and honesty by doctors and hospitals, explaining to them that when they hide and stonewall, they make new victims out of not only family members but also the health-care providers themselves. As she wrote recently, "Without practicing disclosure and transparency, you are burying, with our family members, the very answers to some of the most important questions that will lead you to some of the answers for your most daunting problems."[5]

Nancy's lesson for families who have experienced an injury in a hospital or clinic is never to give up on finding out what happened. It will help you, but more important, it will help the next patient. The life you save, if not your own, may be someone else's.

Peter Pronovost: Doctor, Champion—and Promoter of the Lifesaving Checklist

Peter Pronovost, a recipient of one of the Pete Conrad awards, looks young enough to need to show ID to buy a drink but is actually in his midforties. Dr. Pronovost, whom we met in Chapters 12 and 13, is director of the Center for Innovation in Quality Patient Care at Johns Hopkins University in Baltimore. He bubbles with enthusiasm and ideas, and he has proven, in the pages of leading journals like the *New England Journal of Medicine,* that simple innovations can save lives: for instance, his checklist for inserting central lines. He has both a PhD in medical research and an MD, and he is board certified in intensive care and anesthesiology. So Peter Pronovost is way beyond most of us lay folks in his technical medical sophistication. Yet Pronovost too, like the other patient advocates featured in this chapter, became involved with the patient safety movement because of a tragedy in his own family.

Peter was in his fourth year of medical school at Hopkins when, in 1991, he returned to his Connecticut home to help his father in his last days. Henry Pronovost, a mathematics teacher in a community college, was only fifty-one years old. He had a lymph-gland cancer that had been misdiagnosed as a blood cancer; the window of opportunity for a cure closed before the correct diagnosis was made. That was one mistake, but not the last. "I carried his crumbling eighty-pound body up to a bed in our home," Peter recalled in an interview with me. "He was going to die with hospice. For the next week as he was dying, he writhed in pain, and our pleas to the hospice staff were met with 'nothing we can do.' As I became a doctor, I realized this was wrong. I realized we needed to do better."

Now, Peter's institute at Hopkins is pushing forward several pilot projects for patient safety, including the "safe surgery" checklist that was adopted by the World Health Organization (see Chapter 11). Medicine has plenty of guidelines for best practices, but they tend to go on for dozens, even hundreds of pages. The checklist idea, which was borrowed from aviation safety, starts with boiling down the key recommendations into short lists that people can remember.

In making the checklist work, says Pronovost, right behind simplicity is humility, the realization that doctors don't know everything, that they need to use simple checklists, and that nurses and even patients have a right to police their work and make sure the right things are done.

I asked Pronovost for a checklist of what patients and their families should do. Here's what he said:

1. First, be inquisitive. People should be really comfortable advocating and questioning about what happens to their own bodies. Patients need to speak up and ask questions and understand, and if the hospitals and doctors aren't interested in being questioned, that should be a huge red flag.
2. Know your medicines. Know why you're taking them and how you're supposed to take them.
3. Know what procedure you're going in for, so you don't get the wrong one.
4. Advocate for safety when doctors and nurses come in your room. They should wash their hands every time before they touch you.
5. Every day in the hospital, ask what today's goals are. Find out what is preventing you from going home and how they're going to work on it today.
6. When you leave the hospital, be very comfortable and clear on what is supposed to happen next.

Pronovost also wants patients to advocate politically for full disclosure of things like infection rates. As we've seen in Chapter 14 on choosing a hospital, the information out there now is spotty and hard to understand. Pronovost says that hospitals now can make noble statements on their Web sites about quality and safety, but consumers cannot verify their truth "because there are no standards about how to gather and evaluate the safety data." The voluntary, inconsistent disclosure practices now prevalent in the industry need to give way to mandatory, uniform standards.

I have borrowed Peter Pronovost's "checklist" ideas throughout this book—short lists of key questions you need to ask to make sure you and your family get the right care. But the key lesson that Pronovost teaches, I think, is to have the right attitude: He tells doctors and nurses to be humble, and patients to be inquisitive, and to speak up.

Beth McGlynn: Researcher, Champion—She Proved That Low Quality Is Everybody's Problem

You might not guess it from Beth McGlynn's careful, dry prose, or from her business suits and tight auburn curls, or from her PhD in public policy, but she is really a health-care revolutionary at heart. Or at least a radical reformer. McGlynn has headed a team from the RAND think tank in a decade-long project to measure and document the quality of care that all kinds of Americans receive for all kinds of diseases: rich and poor, educated and not, insured and uninsured, from California to Maine, Minnesota to Florida. Her team has issued a series of report cards with an emperor-is-wearing-no-clothes message: No matter who you are, or where you live, you are at high risk of receiving poor-quality health care.

Denial is a major focus of McGlynn's work. Everybody thinks that the problem of mediocre and poor health care may happen to somebody else, but not to them. Their own care, many people think, is pretty good. McGlynn's work proves scientifically that we're all at high risk of poor care. First, her group randomly sampled patients in twelve metropolitan areas across the country and found that, overall, patients received about half of the recommended care on the quality indicators list.[6] Care for chronic illnesses, acute ailments, and preventive care all got about the same level of mediocrity. Treatment of eye cataracts and breast cancer got the highest marks, above 75 percent, while alcohol dependence was the worst performer, with only 10 percent of the recommended care being given.

Well, this doesn't apply to me, I can hear you thinking, *because I have insurance and make a good income.* Think again. The RAND group studied those variables and found that they matter, but not much. People with household incomes under $15,000 got about 53 percent of the recommended care, while those with incomes over

$50,000 got 56 percent of the recommended care, no real difference at all. They also found that women versus men, and blacks and Hispanics versus whites, had some similarly slight differences in care quality, but again, not much. These were published in a follow-up report.[7] There was some regional variation too, but piddling: People in Seattle, the highest-scoring city, got 59 percent of recommended care, versus 51 percent in Little Rock, Arkansas, the lowest-scoring city. Where I went to school, 59 percent is a flunking grade and not much to brag about compared to 51 percent.

The lesson from these numbers, says Beth McGlynn, is that if you think you're getting good care because you just assume so, chances are you're wrong. The system, she says, is frighteningly random: "It's not really a system; it's just not organized to match up your unique needs with the care you need." So I asked McGlynn how she deals with the randomness of health-care quality in her own life and what she recommends to friends and family. I already quoted her in Chapter 3 on talking to your doctor, about her use of an index-card list of talking points when she goes to her primary doctor. Here's what else she says:

"I really think it's important to find a doctor that you can talk to and they listen. My doctor listens and takes me seriously. That's one of the reasons I stick with her. If you talk to doctors who are superb diagnosticians, they tell you that the patient has all the information they need for the diagnosis. So this is a relationship you need to make work. If it doesn't work, you have to go to someone else whom you're not afraid to talk to. In hospitals when we look at what goes wrong, it's almost always a failure of communications."

Intimidation is another huge problem, as we've talked about throughout this book. McGlynn tells the story of her father, a retired hospital administrator, who despite his lifelong career in health care, was afraid to talk to his doctor about his heart medications that weren't working. He was halfway across the country and McGlynn couldn't advocate in person for him, but she prevailed on a doctor she knew to write out a review of the medications; she faxed it to her dad, and that gave him the weapon he needed to talk to the doctor. Her conclusion: "When you can't advocate for yourself, you have to have someone else do it for you."

McGlynn also recommends some other questions for the doctor: "What can I do to avoid surgery?" And: "This test you want me to have, how will its result change the treatment plan?" (If it doesn't, that's a good reason to skip the test.)

Finally, she says, "I'm really committed to making the health-care system better so people don't have to worry about what hospital or what doctor to go to. I don't want people to have to advocate for their own care. But we're a ways from there, a good ways."

Which is exactly why I wrote this book. For those readers now brimming with good health, but who also have a realistic appraisal of what lies ahead, who have no time to wait for health-care reform, and who want to stretch the horizon of life to its natural healthy limit, the nine steps I advocate will help ensure that the life you save will be your own.

Epilogue: Dealing With Medical Injury

The doctor said my friend Steve Massey's rectal bleeding was from hemorrhoids—nothing to worry about. It turned out to be colon cancer. A widow told me how she had taken her husband to the emergency room after he woke up with terrible chest pain. The doctors said it was indigestion from something he ate and sent them home. Two hours later, he was dead on the kitchen floor with a heart attack—the bottle of Maalox near his outstretched hand.

My friend Steve and my client were among the hundreds of thousands of patients injured and killed every year by preventable medical error and poor-quality care. If it happens to you or a loved one, this is my book's final advice on what to do.

First, in fairness to the doctors and nurses involved, you have to hold out the possibility that a reasonable explanation exists for what happened. But you have to politely insist on hearing that explanation—or whatever the truth is.

There are many clues. When a routine illness turns into disaster without warning, when doctors abruptly turn defensive and uncommunicative—these are the signs that sometimes make patients and their families start to ask difficult questions about the quality of the medical care.

How to proceed is a delicate and difficult task. Like most people, if something has taken an unexpected turn for the worse, you want to know why. But you don't want to alienate caregivers who still might be important to ongoing care.

The best way to proceed is to follow some simple, logical steps.

Step One:
Ask the caregivers non-judgmental questions about what happened.

Your first step is to find out what happened. As Joe Friday said, "Just the facts, ma'am." This is not the time to make judgments. There will be time for that later.

You don't necessarily have to confront the main caregiver whom you fear has caused an injury. In most hospital settings, there are numerous doctors and nurses who are knowledgeable about the case and can fill in at least part of the picture. Ask them what they know. If they don't know, ask them:

- Who else should I talk to?
- Do they recommend any Internet research, books, articles, etc., which can help you understand the situation?

What if they won't talk to you, or speak only in generalities, or technicalities that you can't understand? Here's where it helps to know your rights. The patient (or the patient's representatives if the patient is incapacitated) has an absolute right to know what has happened to them. You can read it right in the American Medical Association Code of Medical Ethics, section 8.12, which is worth reprinting in full (I've italicized some of the key language):

> It is a fundamental ethical requirement that a physician should at all times deal honestly and openly with patients. Patients have a right to know their past and present medical status and to be free of any mistaken beliefs concerning their conditions. Situations occasionally occur in which a patient suffers significant medical complications that may have resulted from the physician's mistake or judgment. In these situations, *the physician is ethically required to inform the patient of all the facts necessary to ensure understanding of what has occurred.* Only through full disclosure is a patient able to make informed decisions regarding future medical care. Ethical responsibility includes informing patients of changes in their diagnoses resulting from retrospective review of test results or any other information. This obligation holds even though the patient's medical treatment or therapeutic options may not be altered by the new information. *Concern regarding legal liability which might result following truthful disclosure should not affect the physician's honesty with a patient.*
>
> —Issued March 1981; updated June 1994.

More recently, the AMA has backed off this noble ethical position with a new statement that shows more concern for doctors' legal liability: ethics section 8.121, issued in December 2003, states in part,

> When patient harm has been caused by an error, physicians should offer a *general explanation* regarding the nature of the error and the measures being taken to prevent similar occurrences in the future. Such communication is fundamental to the trust that underlies the patient-physician relationship, and may help reduce the risk of liability. [Emphasis added.]

A "general explanation," of course, could turn out to be so broad and vague that it is no explanation at all. But the old ethical provision, section 8.12, is still on the AMA's books and is worth calling to the attention of health-care providers who refuse to be informative.

Some doctors argue that they should not have to explain anything to patients that could land them in a lawsuit. A few state legislatures have responded with laws that protect anything a doctor says by way of apology or explanation from being used against the doctor in court. But how sincere is an apology when it is offered under such a legal cloak of protection? Other health-care providers, notably the Veterans Administration Hospital in Lexington, Kentucky, have adopted a policy of full disclosure and let the chips fall where they may. The Lexington Veterans Hospital found that patients appreciate the candor and are no more likely to sue than at other hospitals where patients find it harder to learn the facts. [1]

Step Two:
Ask the hospital to investigate.

You can ask the hospital to do its own investigation, especially if the injury is particularly serious. You may meet someone called the hospital "risk manager." The "risks" they manage are mainly risks of lawsuits, and only secondarily risks to patient safety. So once the risk manager is involved, you may not learn much useful information. Unfortunately the official results of any hospital investigation are protected by law in most states from disclosure to patients or their lawyers. However, you can expect at least *some* explanation will be forthcoming from the hospital's official investigation, so it might be worth trying.

Bear in mind that many hospitals—shamed by the stories of patients like Sue Sheridan and Nancy Conrad, which we talked about in the last chapter—now have adopted a disclosure mandate that requires them to reveal to the patient when a "never event" has occurred.

Every now and then (a lot less often than it should happen), a hospital will actually admit error and try to offer you a settlement to avoid a lawsuit. You will need a lawyer to help you evaluate the fairness of the hospital's offer and negotiate the best settlement for you. That lawyer should work at a much discounted rate to the usual contingency fee, which assumes a risk of zero recovery. If the hospital tries to get you to settle without going to a lawyer, that's a red flag that you're about to be taken advantage of; this is not something that ethical hospitals do.

Step Three:
Ask for an independent investigation by a health-care-quality agency.

Your choices here are limited. It's a waste of time to ask the local or state medical society to investigate. They have no power to do anything and are likely to side with the providers. (But sometimes the medical society will have a reasonably honest mediation service for billing disputes through an ethics committee.[2])

The Joint Commission, which is a joint project of various medical and hospital private associations, will investigate a quality of care complaint but won't tell you the results. Go to http://www.jointcommission.org. To its credit, though, the Joint Commission has a rule for hospitals it accredits that *requires* them to disclose to patients any harmful medical error that has occurred to them. (The problem is that only a few brave pioneering institutions have realized that honesty is always the best policy.)

These government agencies investigate complaints of poor-quality health care:

- The state or local health department can investigate outbreaks of infection to find if proper sterilization procedures were followed. Unfortunately most health departments have no ability to go beyond infections to other issues, nor do they have the manpower or expertise.

- The state licensing board has the power to revoke or suspend any health-care provider's license. But this is done typically only in egregious circumstances, such as illegal drug use or other criminal behavior. Most boards are grossly understaffed and unequipped to deal with ordinary negligence or carelessness that hurts patients. You can find a list of licensing boards at the umbrella organization for licensing boards: the National Board of Medical Examiners, http://www.nbme.org.
- The local Medicare Quality Improvement Organization (QIO). Never heard of it? Most people haven't. But these groups, which were set up by Congress and funded by the taxpayers to improve the quality of care given to Medicare beneficiaries, have the muscle to get to the bottom of incidents in hospitals. And patients have a right to find out what the QIO learned.

How do you prod the Medicare QIO to investigate? A Medicare beneficiary, or someone acting on the beneficiary's behalf, must file a written complaint. The subject of the complaint has to concern "the quality of services . . . not meeting professionally recognized standards of health care." (The statute is 42 U.S.C. § 1320c-3(a)(14).) Go to this Web site for a list of QIOs: http://www.qualitynet.org. There is one for each state.[3]

Thanks to a lawsuit brought against the federal government by Public Citizen, you have a right to learn the results of any investigation done by a QIO. The Court of Appeals for the D.C. Circuit ruled that: "At a minimum, this means that the [QIO] must disclose its determination as to whether the quality of the services that the recipient received met 'professionally recognized standards of health care.'"[4]

There are two issues here. Why hire a lawyer? And what lawyer to hire?

Step Four:
Hire a lawyer—but not just any lawyer.

Why Hire a Lawyer?

However candid or guarded the health-care providers appear to be in your dealings with them, there is only one way to get to the bottom of whether malpractice has occurred. That is to have the treatment evaluated by expert physicians of the same specialty with no connection to the treating doctors.

If you have medical connections among your family or friends, you can try to do this on your own. Usually, though, people turn to lawyers to advise them and act as go-betweens in obtaining independent evaluation. The good news is that there are many highly competent lawyers who will do this initial investigation for you without charging for their time.

It takes time to find the right lawyer and obtain the best advice. This can be frustrating, but in the long run, it's best to go slow. Rushing into a lawsuit when one is still feeling shock and anger is usually unwise. Lawsuits can linger for years and involve maddening uncertainty. Worse, the legal process forces a victim to relive the experience over and over in microscopic detail.

A careful study beforehand helps to ensure that the decision to sue—or more often, not to sue—is the right one.

The evaluative process starts with acquiring copies of all the pertinent medical records. You can expect to be asked to sign a number of release forms, which the lawyer will then use to request the records. This often means contacting half a dozen or more doctors and hospitals for office notes, X-ray films, lab tests, and other pertinent data.

Then the lawyer must find the right specialist to go over the records. Sometimes the expert will want to see the patient; more often a good preliminary evaluation can be made from the records supplemented by well-focused statements from the patient and family members about the chronology of key symptoms and treatment events.

The expert looks at the case with two questions in mind:

- Did the care violate established standards of practice?
- Did the care make a significant difference in worsening the patient's health?

If the answer to either or both questions is no, there is no malpractice case. And that is the usual situation. Experienced medical malpractice lawyers report that nine out of ten times, they ultimately tell the family that there is no case—even where circumstances at first suggested serious wrongdoing.

This reality is at odds with the common myth that lawyers will encourage meritless suits in hopes of scoring a quick settlement from the insurance company. The fact is that companies insuring doctors and hospitals fight claims doggedly, both meritorious ones and those without merit. Industry statistics show that more than half of all malpractice claims are closed with no payout to the patient, and of cases that go to trial, doctors win about 70 percent.

That is why good malpractice lawyers, whose fee is nothing if they lose, pick and choose their cases carefully.

What Lawyer to Hire?

How do you find a good lawyer to make the initial study of the case? It's hard enough to find a good doctor—and there you have plenty of word-of-mouth advice from friends about doctors they have dealt with. Few if any of your friends will have experience with a subspecialty like medical malpractice lawyers.

You might turn to the Yellow Pages. In contrast to the gray pages of the physicians' section of the telephone book, you will find page after page of bold-faced headlines from attorneys who claim to handle medical malpractice cases. Many of the ads specify the type of injuries these lawyers are most interested in: "death," "brain damage," "quadriplegia"—a litany of the worst injuries people can suffer, and not coincidentally, the most lucrative injuries for lawyers on a contingent fee based on a percentage of the final settlement or jury verdict. Some even tell you they make house calls.

Some of these lawyers are excellent. Others are not. And some of the best lawyers don't advertise at all. Finding the best takes work. A good place to start is by contacting any lawyers you know (a friendly judge would be an even better source) who do not handle personal injury cases. Who would they go to if it were a member of their own family?

Directories of lawyers are available online and in any library. The most comprehensive is called *Martindale-Hubbell Law Directory*. Look for articles the lawyer has written, awards from fellow lawyers, and other signs that make the lawyer stand out from the crowd. Sooner or later you will find yourself in the lawyer's office. Be sure to ask about recent verdicts and current cases to find out whether he or she is currently active—and successful—or whether the claim to expertise is based on past and faded glories. Ask about his or her experience in cases like yours. A lawyer who has handled cases involving falls out of hospital beds is not necessarily equipped for complicated obstetric cases.

Beware of lawyers who are eager to sign you to a contingent-fee contract with them before they have evaluated the merits of your case. This lawyer will often want to bail out when he has failed to get a quick—and usually cheap—settlement with the insurance company. Or if he is really incompetent, he will run up thousands of dollars in expenses that you are obligated to pay in pursuit of a marginal and ultimately worthless claim.

Personality is obviously important too. If the lawyer doesn't listen carefully and patiently to you at your first meeting (when he or she is usually trying to give a good impression), it's not going to get any better.

The evaluation usually costs nothing for the lawyer's time. The lawyer also often absorbs the cost of consulting with an expert, though it is common to ask the client, particularly in an iffy case, to advance five hundred to a thousand dollars or more for the expert's fee.

If the lawyer agrees to take the case, the client will be asked to sign a standard contingent-fee contract. Usually these contracts call for the lawyer to receive one-third of any settlement or verdict, plus expenses of experts, court reporters, and the like. Sometimes clients are asked to pay expenses regularly during the case; other times the lawyer will pay all expenses and deduct them from the final recovery. It is also possible to hire a good lawyer on an hourly fee—the same basis that large companies hire lawyers for commercial litigation. Most clients can't afford this, and even those who can often prefer to share the risk with the lawyer by entering a contingent-fee contract.

What if you sign on with a lawyer and later conclude that he or she is not right for you? It's not hard to fire a lawyer, especially if it's early in the case—although in some cases the lawyer may have a right to hold on to the files of your case until expenses are reimbursed. Sometimes a better option is to ask the lawyer to bring in as cocounsel another more experienced lawyer or law firm. Usually this can be done with no extra charge to the client; the two firms will split the work and divide the eventual contingent fee accordingly.

The bottom line is that the best advice—as in so many situations—is to be careful and ask lots of questions. Are there any questions too stupid to ask? No.

A Final Word on Jury Justice in Malpractice Cases

Here is some sobering news before you venture into the world of lawsuits. The stereotype of the American jury in personal injury cases is the million-dollar award to the lady who spilled hot McDonald's coffee in her lap. The insurance industry has worked hard to promulgate this image of jurors as free-spending, victim-loving, fact-ignoring simpletons. If you buy what they're selling, you're likely to be extra skeptical of any victim if you're called to sit on a jury, just to prove that you're no fool. Which is precisely the point of the propaganda.

And the propaganda works spectacularly well, as study after study has shown. The fact is, victims of malpractice do not get a fair shake from juries, as the insurance industry's own studies have proven.

Seven studies over the past three decades have compared the outcome of jury trials with the private evaluations by the insurance company of their own doctors' performance.[5] The studies have been remarkably consistent: Even where doctor reviewers have rated the medical care "indefensible" or "poor," plaintiffs win at trial no more than 50 percent of the time. When the doctor reviewers have rated the care "defensible," the juries overwhelmingly agree, and vote for the defendant doctors 80 to 90 percent of the time. When different reviewers disagree about the quality of the care, and so the case is rated "unclear" or "a toss-up," the defendants still win around 70 percent of the time. Note the logical pattern in the research: As the evidence of negligence becomes more clear, the victim win rate goes up. But it almost never gets higher than 50 percent, even in the "indefensible" cases. Juries have a very heavy thumb on the scales of justice favoring the doctor defendant.

How are "indefensible" cases defended? For starters, juries never hear about the "indefensible" evaluations. Those are tucked into a very private file back at the insurance company headquarters. A skilled lawyer is hired to defend the case and is set loose to find an expert witness willing to defend the care. Lawyer friends who have done defense work tell me that in an egregious case, it's not uncommon for them to be turned down eight, nine, or more times until they finally find a doctor who will bless the doctor's care. Of course, the jury never hears about the turn-downs. For all the jury can see, the plaintiff has an expert, and the defense has an expert, and they're both pretty glib, and so the benefit of the doubt goes to the doctor, who, after all, was only trying to help his patient.

I mention these studies here for two reasons: It underscores the importance of hiring a top attorney if a lawsuit is your only option, and it shows why you and your family are so much better off following the nine necessary steps I have set out in this book to win the best care for yourselves so you never face the prospect of having to file suit.

Acknowledgments

The people whose stories populate this book have let me relate some of the most harrowing, difficult, and even humiliating episodes of their lives. Some preferred anonymity; others allowed me to identify them, and you will find their names throughout this book. To all of them, anonymous and named, I offer thanks for their generous sharing.

Research assistance came from Sabrina Kang, Anjali Bhat, Janice Toliver, Leonard Dooren, Ciara Malone, and Andrea Shrieves.

My editor, Renée Sedliar, helped me to broaden the book's focus; she gave valuable insights at all stages of writing.

Several physicians generously read all or parts of the manuscript and offered valuable insights, corrections, and guidance. They include Dr. Mark Hoffman (also an accomplished attorney), Dr. David Shapiro, Dr. Tom Masterson, Dr. Joy Lewis, and especially, Dr. Andy Thomson. All errors remain mine alone.

Other health-care professionals who submitted to interviews and otherwise gave valuable help include Dr. Peter Pronovost, Dr. Beth

McGlynn of the RAND Institute, Betsy McCaughey, Jim Conway of the Institute for Healthcare Improvement, Matt Austin of the Leapfrog Group, Dr. Ashish Jha of Harvard, and Angela Neumeyer-Gromen of the Max Planck Institute for Human Development.

Two excellent lawyers led me to patients willing to share the stories of their encounters with the health-care system: Robert Spohrer of Jacksonville, Florida, and Roger Pardieck of Seymour, Indiana. Thanks also to Jim Bostwick, a fine San Francisco lawyer, for his thoughts. My sons Ian and Chris Malone and my friend David Stewart gave helpful advice as well.

Resources and Further Reading

Web Sites

The Internet is a vast ocean of information, some of it excellent, some of it misleading and just plain wrong. I have quoted and cited from reliable Web sites throughout this book. Here, I want to highlight a few of the lesser known but noteworthy online resources for patient self-education:

Cancerguide.org: This Web site was started by a cancer patient named Steve Dunn who first thought his kidney cancer would doom him to death in less than a year. He lived many years and died of an infection unrelated to the cancer. He put together this site, which collects highly reliable information from diverse sources. Since his death in 2005, other cancer patients, grateful for his pathbreaking work, have carried on the site on a volunteer basis.

Guidelines.gov: This site is aimed at professionals, so it's a bit technical, but it has a comprehensive compilation of medical practice guidelines for more than 2,000 conditions. It is updated every week by the Agency for Healthcare Research and Quality, a branch of the U.S. Department of Health and Human Services.

Labtestsonline.org: Lab Tests Online lets you look up any lab test and find out why it's given and how to understand your test results. The site is a non-commercial collaboration among professional societies representing the clinical laboratory community, organized by the American Association for Clinical Chemistry.

MedlinePlus (http://www.nlm.nih.gov/medlineplus): MedlinePlus brings together authoritative information from government agencies and private health-care organizations. It was put together by the National Institutes of Health with the National Library of Medicine, which has long operated Medline, the premier search engine for the ever growing universe of medical journal articles from all over the world (16 million articles in 5,200 journals, at last count). Medline itself (accessible at http://www.pubmed.com, can be intimidating for laypersons. MedlinePlus has preformatted Medline searches to help you get started in researching your disease. MedlinePlus also has extensive information about drugs, an illustrated medical encyclopedia, interactive patient tutorials, and health news.

UpToDate.com: This is a noncommercial collaboration that brings together 3,800 top experts in all medical specialties who write, edit, and peer-review a comprehensive set of articles on 7,400 medical topics. Hundreds of these topics written for patients are available free, but for detailed information you have to pay a fee. The big advantages that make the entry fee worth paying are (1) continuous updating, with new research not just thrown into the top of the pile, but placed into context; (2) a grading system that rates the strength of evidence for every treatment recommendation, based on the rigor of research behind it; and (3) top authorities in every field. It's not possible to eliminate all commercial influence from medical advice, but this site tries hard. The site does not accept advertising from drug companies or other commercial interests, and it discloses potential conflicts of interest of its authors at the top of each article.

Blogs

Of the thousands of health-care-related blogs, one stands out to me as having the most consistently interesting and literate entries: Tara Parker-Pope's Well blog at the New York Times site (http://well.blogs.nytimes.com). A special bonus is the high quality of the readers' comments.

I have my own blog, Patient Safety Blog, not nearly as comprehensive, but then this is a part-time labor of love: http://www.protectpatientsblog.com.

Books

Of the many, many books on patient education, I want to single out these as especially noteworthy:

How Doctors Think, by Jerome Groopman, MD (New York: Houghton Mifflin, 2007). Dr. Groopman, a Harvard medical professor and regular contributor to the *New Yorker*, minimizes some of the real horrors of the American health-care system but provides valuable, sophisticated insight into the realities of the diagnostic process and how patients can help steer their doctors in the right direction. I am indebted to Dr. Groopman for articulating the key question, "Doctor, what else could it be?", which informs Chapter 4.

You, the Smart Patient: An Insider's Handbook for Getting the Best Treatment, by Michael Roizen, MD, and Mehmet Oz, MD (New York: Free Press, 2006). The breezy tone and the cartoons may annoy you, but this book is a worthy read, crammed with good advice.

Calculated Risks: How to Know When Numbers Deceive You, by Gerd Gigerenzer (New York: Simon & Schuster, 2002). Dr. Gigerenzer, who is a professor at the Harding Center for Risk Literacy at the Max Planck Institute for Human Development in Berlin, Germany, brings home with elegant examples the importance of patients learning to be literate with statistics.

Medical Abbreviations: 30,000 Conveniences at the Expense Of Communication and Safety, 14th ed., by Neil M. Davis (Warminster, PA: Neil M. Davis

Associates, 2008). Davis, a Pennsylvania pharmacist, has campaigned for decades to reduce the proliferation of abbreviations in the medical industry because they create dangerous ambiguities and misunderstandings. His book started with a few hundred abbreviations and seems to mushroom with each edition. The book is arranged in alphabetical order so you can see for yourself why, for example, "OD," which means both "once daily" and "right eye," has resulted in medications being wrongly administered to the right eye. But on the most practical level, his book is invaluable for deciphering your own medical records.

Appendix A: Twenty-eight Things That Should Never Happen in a Health-Care Facility

This list is reprinted with permission from the National Quality Forum's list, "Serious Reportable Events in Healthcare."* Explanations in brackets are mine, not the National Quality Forum's.

1. **Surgical Events**
   A. Surgery performed on the wrong body part
   B. Surgery performed on the wrong patient
   C. Wrong surgical procedure performed on a patient
   D. Unintended retention of a foreign object in a patient after surgery or other procedure

*This list is amplified—with explanations and exceptions—in the National Quality Forum's "Serious Reportable Events in Health Care—2006 Update," accessible at http://www.qualityforum.org/pdf/reports/sre/txsrepublic.pdf.

E. Intra-operative or immediately postoperative death in an ASA Class I patient [American Society of Anesthesiologists system rating the health of patients going into a surgery; class I patients are completely healthy.]

2. **Product or Device Events**
   A. Patient death or serious disability associated with the use of contaminated drugs, devices, or biologics provided by the healthcare facility
   B. Patient death or serious disability associated with the use or function of a device in patient care in which the device is used for functions other than as intended
   C. Patient death or serious disability associated with intravascular air embolism [an air bubble in the bloodstream] that occurs while being cared for in a healthcare facility

3. **Patient Protection Events**
   A. Infant discharged to the wrong person
   B. Patient death or serious disability associated with patient elopement (disappearance)
   C. Patient suicide, or attempted suicide, resulting in serious disability while being cared for in a healthcare facility

4. **Care Management Events**
   A. Patient death or serious disability associated with a medication error (e.g., errors involving the wrong drug, wrong dose, wrong patient, wrong time, wrong rate, wrong preparation, or wrong route of administration)
   B. Patient death or serious disability associated with a hemolytic reaction due to the administration of ABO/HLA-incompatible blood or blood products [Blood cells self-destruct because the blood transfused into a patient is not the same type as the patient's blood.]
   C. Maternal death or serious disability associated with labor or delivery in a low-risk pregnancy while being cared for in a healthcare facility

D. Patient death or serious disability associated with hypoglycemia [low blood sugar], the onset of which occurs while the patient is being cared for in a healthcare facility

E. Death or serious disability (kernicterus) associated with failure to identify and treat hyperbilirubinemia in neonates [Kernicterus is a brain injury that happens in newborns when their bodies do not process bile properly, so an excess amount of bilirubin, the key component of bile, builds up in the blood. It is considered totally preventable; treatments include shining strong lights on the baby's skin or, in some cases, giving blood transfusions. See Sue Sheridan's story in the final chapter.]

F. Stage 3 or 4 pressure ulcers acquired after admission to a healthcare facility [Also known as bedsores, these are wounds caused by a bedridden patient not being moved enough; stage 3 and 4 are the worst stages, where the wound extends down to the bone. See discussion in Chapter 12, page 157.]

G. Patient death or serious disability due to spinal manipulative therapy [chiropractic treatment]

H. Artificial insemination with the wrong donor sperm or wrong egg

5. **Environmental Events**

A. Patient death or serious disability associated with an electric shock while being cared for in a healthcare facility

B. Any incident in which a line designated for oxygen or other gas to be delivered to a patient contains the wrong gas or is contaminated by toxic substances

C. Patient death or serious disability associated with a burn incurred from any source while being cared for in a healthcare facility

D. Patient death or serious disability associated with a fall while being cared for in a healthcare facility

E. Patient death or serious disability associated with the use of restraints or bedrails while being cared for in a healthcare facility

6. **Criminal Events**
   A. Any instance of care ordered by or provided by someone impersonating a physician, nurse, pharmacist, or other licensed healthcare provider
   B. Abduction of a patient of any age
   C. Sexual assault on a patient within or on the grounds of the healthcare facility
   D. Death or significant injury of a patient or staff member resulting from a physical assault (i.e., battery) that occurs within or on the grounds of the healthcare facility

Appendix B: High-Risk Situations in Biopsy Diagnosis of Cancer

If you're not totally convinced that *any* and *every* biopsy deserves a second look, here is a list from a surgical pathologist of high-risk situations, which deserve a closer look every single time.

1. **Breast biopsies** with diagnoses of atypical ductal hyperplasia and ductal carcinoma in situ
2. **D&Cs (uterine scrapings)** that are diagnosed as atypical hyperplasia, dysplasia, or borderline hyperplasia, especially on several occurrences
3. **Prostate biopsies** that show high-grade atypia, particularly on multiple occasions
4. **Pigmented (dark-colored) mole or birthmark** that was removed because of suspicion of malignant melanoma (a type of skin cancer) and skin lesions that are called borderline melanoma or atypical melanocytic hyperplasia

5. **Lymph-node biopsies** with any of the following diagnoses: atypical lymphoid hyperplasia, non-Hodgkins lymphoma, and Hodgkins lymphoma (Hodgkins disease)
6. **Soft-tissue** or **bone tumors** (sarcomas)
7. **Cancer that has spread (metastasized)** but the primary site (organ in which the cancer began) cannot be determined
8. Any **unusual** or **rare** kinds of cancer
9. **Colon biopsies** from patients with ulcerative colitis that show atypia or dysplasia
10. **Esophagus biopsies** in patients with Barrett's esophagus that are diagnosed with high-grade dysplasia
11. Biopsies described in the pathology report as "**worrisome**," "**suspicious**," or "**borderline**"

I can testify from my own experience as a patient advocate that too often what is "borderline" or "atypical" to one pathologist is obvious cancer to a more experienced pathologist.

Appendix C: Fifteen Steps You Can Take to Reduce Your Risk of a Hospital Infection*

From the Committee to Reduce Infection Deaths

Most of us will have to go into the hospital someday. Here are specific steps you can follow to protect yourself from deadly hospital infections:

1. **Ask that hospital staff clean their hands before treating you, and ask visitors to clean their hands too.** This is the single most important way to protect yourself in the hospital. If you're worried about being too aggressive, just remember your life could be at stake. All caregivers should clean their hands before treating you. Alcohol-based hand cleaners are more effective at removing most bacteria than soap and water. Do not hesitate to say, "Excuse me, but there's an alcohol dispenser right there. Would you mind using

*©2008, Committee to Reduce Infection Deaths, reprinted with permission, footnotes omitted.

that before you touch me, so I can see it?" Don't be falsely assured by gloves. If caregivers have pulled on gloves without cleaning their hands first, the gloves are already contaminated before they touch you.

2. **Before your doctor uses a stethoscope, ask that the diaphragm (the flat surface) be wiped with alcohol.** Stethoscopes are often contaminated with *Staphylococcus aureus* and other dangerous bacteria, because caregivers seldom take the time to clean them in between patient use.
3. **If you need a "central line" catheter, ask your doctor about the benefits of one that is antibiotic-impregnated or silver-chlorhexidine coated to reduce infections.**
4. **If you need surgery, choose a surgeon with a low infection rate.** Surgeons know their rate of infection for various procedures. Don't be afraid to ask for it.
5. **Beginning three to five days before surgery, shower or bathe daily with chlorhexidine soap.** Various brands can be bought without a prescription. It will help remove any dangerous bacteria you may be carrying on your own skin.
6. **Ask your surgeon to have you tested for methicillin-resistant Staphylococcus aureus (MRSA) at least one week before you come into the hospital.** The test is simple, usually just a nasal swab. If you have it, extra precautions can be taken to protect you from infection.
7. **Stop smoking well in advance of your surgery.** Patients who smoke are three times as likely to develop a surgical site infection as nonsmokers, and have significantly slower recoveries and longer hospital stays.
8. **On the day of your operation, remind your doctor that you may need an antibiotic one hour before the first incision.** For many types of surgery, a presurgical antibiotic is the standard of care, but it is often overlooked by busy hospital staff.
9. **Ask your doctor about keeping you warm during surgery.** Operating rooms are often kept cold, but for many types of surgery, patients who are kept warm resist infection better. This can be done with special blankets, hats, and booties, and warmed IV liquids.

10. **Do not shave the surgical site.** Razors can create small nicks in the skin, through which bacteria can enter. If hair must be removed before surgery, ask that clippers be used instead of a razor.
11. **Avoid touching your hands to your mouth, and do not set food or utensils on furniture or bed sheets.** Germs such as "C. Diff" can live for many days on surfaces and can cause infections if they get into your mouth.
12. **Ask your doctor about monitoring your glucose (sugar) levels continuously during and after surgery, especially if you are having cardiac surgery.** The stress of surgery often makes glucose levels spike erratically. When blood glucose levels are tightly controlled, heart patients resist infection better. Continue monitoring even when you are discharged from the hospital, because you are not fully healed yet.
13. **Avoid a urinary tract catheter if possible.** It is a common cause of infection. The tube allows urine to flow from your bladder out of your body. Sometimes catheters are used when busy hospital staff members don't have time to walk patients to the bathroom. If you have a catheter, ask your caregiver to remove it as soon as possible.
14. **If you must have an IV, make sure that it's inserted and removed under clean conditions and changed every three to four days.** Your skin should be cleaned at the site of insertion, and the person treating you should be wearing clean gloves. Alert hospital staff immediately if any redness appears.
15. **If you are planning to have your baby by Caesarean section,** follow the steps listed above as if you were having any other type of surgery.

Notes

Chapter 1

1. Institute of Medicine, *To Err Is Human: Building a Safer Health System* (Washington, D.C.: National Academy Press, 1999), p. 1.

2. . http://www.ihi.org/IHI/Programs/Campaign/Campaign.htm?TabId=1.

3. Elizabeth McGlynn, et al., "The Quality of Health Care Delivered to Adults in the United States," *New England Journal of Medicine* 348 (June 26, 2003): 2635–2645.

Chapter 2

1. http://distractible.org/2008/08/11/getting-along-part-2-patient-rules/.

2. An excellent discussion of the "familiarity effect" and other impediments to rational decision-making can be found in *Kluge: The Haphazard Construction of the Human Mind* (New York: Houghton Mifflin 2008), by New York University psychologist Gary Marcus.

3. http://hpi.georgetown.edu/privacy/records.html.

4. http://www.myphr.com/your_record/index.asp.

5. http://noedb.org/library/features/the_ultimate_guide_to_taking_control_health_records.

6. The veterans' story is important enough for a whole book, and it has one: Phillip Longman, *Best Care Anywhere, Why VA Health Care Is Better Than Yours* (Sausalito, CA: PoliPointPress, 2007).

Chapter 3

1. Jerome Groopman, *How Doctors Think* (New York: Houghton Mifflin, 2007).

2. Karin Rhodes, et al., "Resuscitating the Physician-Patient Relationship: Emergency Department Communication in an Academic Medical Center," *Annals of Emergency Medicine* 44.3 (Sept. 2004): 262–267.

3. W. Levinson, et al., "Physician-Patient Communication. The Relationship with Malpractice Claims Among Primary Care Physicians and Surgeons," *The Journal of the American Medical Association* 277.7 (Feb. 19, 1997): 553–559.

4. Jane Brody, "Personal Health: On the Same Wavelength with the Doctor," *New York Times*, Dec. 25, 2007, p. D7.

5. Faith Fitzgerald, "I Can't Be Bothered," *Annals of Internal Medicine* 148.4 (Feb. 19, 2008): 317–318.

6. http://well.blogs.nytimes.com/2008/03/17/bothering-your-doctor/?scp=2&sq=faith%20fitzgerald&st=cse.

Chapter 5

1. American College of Physicians, "American College of Physicians Ethics Manual. Third Edition," *Annals of Internal Medicine* 117.11 (Dec. 1, 1992): 956.

2. The meeting in 2007 was sponsored by the Mayo Clinic Health Policy Forum and was cohosted by the RAND Corporation. See http://www.mayoclinic.org/healthpolicycenter/forum3-summary.html.

3. http://en.wikipedia.org/wiki/Medical_home.

4. You can look up the full list of the twenty-four specialties and the more than one hundred subspecialties at the ABMS Web site: http://abms.org/.

5. https://www.abms.org/WC/NameAndLocationSearch.aspx.

6. See, for example, the American College of Osteopathic Internists, at http://www.acoi.org.

7. http://www.abim.org/.

8. This quote is taken from Dr. Lamberts's blog, which has much other valuable information for building a sound doctor-patient relationship. See http://distractible.org/2008/08/06/getting-along-part-1-doctor-rules/ and http://distractible.org/2008/08/11/getting-along-part-2-patient-rules/.

Chapter 6

1. http://msspnexus.blogs.com/mspblog/2006/05/dr_john_anderso.html.

2. See http://www.citizen.org/publications/release.cfm?ID7580.

Chapter 7

1. The latest in a series of scandals about hidden payments from the drug industry to medical leaders involves the overpresciption of powerful antipsychotic drugs for teenagers. As documented by Gardiner Harris of the *New York Times*, investigators working for Iowa senator Charles Grassley have turned up case after case of prominent child psychiatrists who promoted these drugs without revealing their large industry payments. See, for example, "Radio Host Has Drug Industry Ties," *New York Times*, Nov. 21, 2008, accessible at http://www.nytimes.com/2008/11/22/health/22radio.html?_r=1.

2. Gregory D. Curfman, Stephen Morrissey, and Jeffrey M. Drazen, "Why Doctors Should Worry About Preemption," *New England Journal of Medicine* 359.1 (July 3, 2008): 1-3.

3. (New York: Random House, 2004).

4. (New York: Bloomsbury, 2007).

5. http://nofreelunch.org/doctors.asp.

6. These and other data in this section come from a report about the study by Tara Parker-Pope in her excellent Well blog at the *New York Times*: http://www.nytimes.com/2008/11/18/health/18well.html?_r=1&scp=3&sq=statins%20CRP&st=cse.

7. See the whole list at Public Citizen's Worst Pills, Best Pills Web site: http://www.worstpills.org/public/page.cfm?op_id=45#10_rules. For a small annual fee, you can search the site for information about specific drugs.

8. http://www.worstpills.org/public/drugsheet.pdf.

Chapter 8

1. The statistics in this and the following paragraph are borrowed from *Calculated Risks: How to Know When Numbers Deceive You* (New York: Simon and Schuster, 2002), by Gerd Gigerenzer, to whom I am indebted. See especially pages 41 to 46.

2. Two more terms go hand-in-glove with false positives and false negatives. They are sensitivity and specificity. The odds that a test will catch people who actually have the disease being tested for is the test's "sensitivity"—the same as its "true positive" rate. The sum of the sensitivity rate and the false-negative rate is always one. So if a test has a 1 percent false-negative rate, it has a sensitivity of 99 percent.

Specificity is the term for when a test catches only people who have the disease, not something else. Specificity is the same as a test's "true negative" rate. A highly specific test will have a low false-alarm (false-positive) rate. The sum of the false-positive rate and the specificity rate for any test is always one (for example, when the false positive rate is 10 percent, the specificity rate is 90 percent). You will often hear doctors say that such and such a test is very "nonspecific," or has a low specificity rate; that means the test generates a lot of false positives.

3. The statistics in this paragraph are borrowed from Gerd Gigerenzer's book, *Calculated Risks: How to Know When Numbers Deceive You* (New York: Simon and Schuster, 2002): 124-126.

4. This is called the paradox of the false positive. Whenever any test generates a higher rate of false positives than the incidence of the disease being tested for in the target population, the positive results from the test are likely to be wrong. See http://en.wikipedia.org/wiki/False_positive_paradox.

5. This discussion is adapted from *Calculated Risks*. Professor Gigerenzer's data is drawn from the National Institutes of Health and the Ontario [Canada] Cancer Registry.

6. http://www.nhlbi.nih.gov/health/hearttruth/press/infograph_leading causes.pdf.

7. Statistics in this paragraph are from *Calculated Risks*, pages 59 to 62.

8. For more on this, read the guidelines from the American College of Physicians on routine mammograms in women in their forties: Amir Qaseem, et al., "Clinical Efficacy Assessment Subcommittee of the Ameri-

can College of Physicians. Screening Mammography for Women Forty to Forty-Nine Years of Age: A Clinical Practice Guideline from the American College of Physicians," *Annals of Internal Medicine* 146.7 (Apr. 3, 2007): 511–515. The full text can be found at http://www.guidelines.gov, a very useful Web site from the U.S. Department of Health and Human Services that lists clinical-practice guidelines for more than 2,000 topics.

Chapter 9

1. http://www.sciencedaily.com/releases/2006/11/061129151415.htm.

2. J. D. Kronz, W. H Westra, and J. I. Epstein, "Mandatory Second Opinion Surgical Pathology at a Large Referral Hospital," *Cancer* 86.11 (December, 1999): 2426–2435.

3. D. Gupta and L. J. Layfield, "Prevalence of Inter-Institutional Anatomic Pathology Slide Review," *The American Journal of Surgical Pathology* 24.2 (Feb. 2000): 280–284.

4. A.C. Lind, C. Bewtra, and J. C. Healy, et al., "Prospective Peer Review in Surgical Pathology," *American Journal of Clinical Pathology* 104 (1995): 560–566.

5. Here's a bonus. While you don't have to travel to Washington to receive the services of the AFIP, if you do come to D.C. as a tourist, you should know that in this city stuffed with world-class museums is an obscure but fascinating museum, in the same building with the AFIP. It's called the National Museum of Health and Medicine, which started out as a museum of Civil War medicine and now encompasses a huge collection that includes human embryos at every stage of development, the amputated leg of a notorious Civil War general, artifacts from President Lincoln's assassination, surgical instruments over the centuries, and many other items of medical history.

6. http://www.naic.org/documents/consumer_alert_claim_denials.htm.

7. For the radiologists' perspective, see, for example, B. J. Hillman, "Commentary: Trying to Regulate Imaging Self-Referral Is Like Playing Whack-A-Mole," *American Journal of Roentgenology* 189.2 (August 2007): 267–268. The full text is accessible at http://www.ajronline.org/cgi/content/full/189/2/267.

8. Reed Abelson, "Cleveland Clinic Discloses Doctors' Industry Ties," *New York Times*, Dec. 2, 2008, accessible at http://www.nytimes.com/2008/12/03/business/03clinic.html?_r=1&ref=business.

Chapter 10

1. http://www.medscape.com/viewarticle/439159_1.

2. You can look up the full list of the twenty-four specialties and the more than one hundred subspecialties at the ABMS Web site: http://abms.org/.

3. Quoted in Michael Levenson and Matt Viser, "Kennedy Has 'Successful' Surgery," *Boston Globe*, June 3, 2008, accessible at http://www.boston.com/news/local/massachusetts/articles/2008/06/03/kennedy_has_successful_surgery/

4. Adapted from Atul A. Gawande, et al., "The Incidence and Nature of Surgical Adverse Events in Colorado and Utah in 1992," *Surgery* 126.1 (July 1999): 66–75, table III.

Chapter 11

1. http://www.startribune.com/lifestyle/health/16769816.html.

2. http://www.independent.ie/national-news/hospital-investigates-botched-removal-of-childs-wrong-kidney-1353861.html.

3. http://www.legalradar.com/2006/06/malpractice_sui.html.

4. http://news.bbc.co.uk/1/hi/wales/2049839.stm.

5. http://www5.aaos.org/wrong/setup.cfm.

6. Implementation Manual for the World Health Organization Surgical Safety Checklist (1st edition), available at http://www.who.int/patientsafety/safesurgery/tools_resources/SSSL_Manual_finalJun08.pdf.

7. Alex Haynes, et al., "A Surgical Safety Checklist to Reduce Morbidity and Mortality in a Global Population," *New England Journal of Medicine* 360.5 (2009): 491–499.

Chapter 12

1. The statistics are from the U.S. Centers for Disease Control and Prevention. A useful factsheet with prevention tips can be found at http://www.cdc.gov/ncipc/factsheets/adultfalls.htm.

2. http://www.chestnet.org/about/awareness/DVTfacts.php.

3. You can see Dr. Caprini's list at http://www.crmhealthcare.net/docs/67450a_CapriniRiskAssessmentTool.pdf.

Chapter 13

1. John Boyce and Didier Pittet, "Guidelines for Hand Hygiene in Health-Care Settings. Recommendations of the Healthcare Infection Control Practices Advisory Committee and the HICPAC/SHEA/APIC/IDSA Hand Hygiene Task Force," *Morbidity and Mortality Weekly Report* 51 (October 25, 2002), available at http://www.cdc.gov/mmwr/preview/mmwrhtml/rr5116a1.htm.

2. Ibid., page 23 and table 8. This table summarizes thirty-four studies done between 1981 and 2000 that showed hand hygiene compliance by health-care workers ranged from 5 percent to 81 percent, with an average of 40 percent.

3. Ibid., at page 23 and box 1.

4. See http://www.consumersunion.org/campaigns/stophospitalinfections/stories.html.

5. Betsy McCaughey, "Unnecessary Deaths: The Human and Financial Costs of Hospital Infections," Committee to Reduce Infection Deaths (3rd edition, 2008, available at http://www.hospitalinfection.org/ridbooklet.pdf) at page 3. Because there is no mandated reporting, health-care experts have to guess at the total number of hospital infections and deaths. Here is the most recent report at the CDC Web site: http://www.cdc.gov/ncidod/dhqp/pdf/hicpac/infections_deaths.pdf.

6. McCaughey, endnotes 18 and 19.

7. More than two-thirds of patient rooms in hospitals are contaminated with MRSA and another deadly drug-resistant bacterium known as VRE. McCaughey, endnotes 21 and 22.

8. The precautions were codified by a group called Society for Healthcare Epidemiology of America (SHEA) in 2003. You can see its twenty-five-page report, with 353 citations, at SHEA's Web site, http://www.shea-online.org/Assets/files/position_papers/SHEA_MRSA_VRE.pdf. SHEA's mission is "to prevent and control infections in health care settings." See http://www.shea-online.org/about/mission.cfm. Unfortunately, that mission does not include telling the public which hospitals follow the "best practices" recommended by SHEA. But I can give you a small sample from scanning the hospital-infection literature of who some of the pioneers in the field are: University of Pittsburgh–Presbyterian Medical Center, Johns Hopkins Hospital and Health Center, Brigham and Women's Hospital in Boston, and the University of Virginia Hospital in Charlottesville, Virginia.

9. This is as of mid-2008. Consumers Union has a state-by-state summary available at http://www.consumersunion.org/campaigns/CU%20Summ%20HAI%20state%20rpting%20laws%20as%20of%201–08.pdf.

10. http://www.consumersunion.org/pdf/MDVAInfections.pdf. The study's authors conclude, "Our analysis shows that the large disparity among hospitals in the same state for trying to prevent infections in surgical patients underscores the need for all consumers in the nation to have access to each hospital's actual rate of infection data. Public reporting of this data will enable patients to choose the best care possible by allowing them to see which hospitals are doing better than others at curbing infection rates. Likewise, it provides incentives to the hospitals and the professionals working there to improve their infection control programs to achieve lower infection rates, therefore improving the quality of patient care."

11. We talked about the role of a bedside advocate in Chapters 3 and 7.

12. Centers for Disease Control and Prevention, *Morbidity and Mortality Weekly Report*, 52 (September 26, 2003). An online report can be found at http://www.cdc.gov/ncidod/dhqp/COCA_Unsafe_Injection_Practices.html.

13. Jane D. Siegel, Emily Rhinehart, Marguerite Jackson, Linda Chiarello, and the Healthcare Infection Control Practices Advisory Committee," 2007 Guideline for Isolation Precautions: Preventing Transmission of Infectious Agents in Healthcare Settings, "Centers for Disease Control and Prevention," June 2007, available at http://www.cdc.gov/ncidod/dhqp/pdf/guidelines/Isolation2007.pdf

14. See http://www.cdc.gov/ncidod/dhqp/injectionsafety.html.

15. http://www.newsday.com/news/local/crime/ny-lidocs265741766jun26,0,710604.story.

16. http://www.newsday.com/news/local/ny-lidocs0624,0,1823319.story.

17. Donald Goldmann, "System Failure Versus Personal Accountability—the Case for Clean Hands," *New England Journal of Medicine* 355.2 (July 13, 2006): 122.

18. All data from J.A. Tan, et al., "Exploring Obstacles to Proper Timing of Prophylactic Antibiotics for Surgical Site Infections," *Quality and Safety in Health Care* 15 (2006): 32–38.

19. Bratzler, "Use of Antimicrobial Prophylaxis for Major Surgery: Baseline Results from the National Surgical Prevention Project," *Archives of Surgery*, 140 (2005): 174–182.

20. J.A. Tan, et al., "Exploring Obstacles to Proper Timing of Prophylactic Antibiotics for Surgical Site Infections," *Quality and Safety in Health Care* 15 (2006): 32–38.

21. http://www.pnhp.org.

Chapter 14

1. The thirty-day rate keeps hospitals from pumping up their survival rates by kicking patients out of the hospital early so that they are recorded as alive when they leave the hospital but then they die soon after.

2. This was a search done on July 6, 2008, at http://www.hospitalcompare.hhs.gov/Hospital/Search/compareHospitals.asp, looking for "hospital outcome of care measures," under "adjusted adult heart attack death rates."

3. This data comes from an interview with Matt Austin of Leapfrog on July 1, 2008.

4. Web site accessed on August 7, 2008.

5. Here's what I found.

Question	Griffin	Yale	Hopkins
Nurses always communicated well	85%	71%	72%
Doctors always communicated well	87%	76%	77%
Always received help as soon as they wanted it	71%	54%	56%
Pain was always well controlled	77%	61%	65%
Staff always explained medications before giving them	72%	53%	57%
Got information about what to do during recovery at home	87%	78%	82%

Chapter 15

1. http://www.turningpointkc.org.

2. http://www.patientslikeme.com/about.

3. Small's story was featured in the *New York Times Magazine*: Thomas Goetz, "Practicing Patients," *New York Times*, March 23, 2008, accessible at http://www.nytimes.com/2008/03/23/magazine/23patients-t.html?emc=eta1.

4. Susan Sontag, *Illness as Metaphor* (New York, Farrar, Strauss & Giroux, 1978).

Chapter 16

1. R. Klein, B.E. Klein, and S.E. Moss, et al., "Glycosylated Hemoglobin Predicts the Incidence and Progression of Diabetic Retinopathy," *Journal of the American Medical Association*, 260 (1988): 2868.

2. F.L. Ferris, "How Effective Are Treatments for Diabetic Retinopathy?" *Journal of the American Medical Association* 269 (1993): 1291.

3. Elizabeth McGlynn, et al., "The Quality of Health Care Delivered to Adults in the United States," *New England Journal of Medicine* 348 (June 26, 2003): 2635-2645; Jinan Saaddine, et al., "A Diabetic Report Card for the United States: Quality of Care in the 1990s," *Annals of Internal Medicine* 136 (2002): 565–574.

4. R. Klein, B.E. Klein, and S.E. Moss, et al., "Glycosylated Hemoglobin Predicts the Incidence and Progression of Diabetic Retinopathy," *Journal of the American Medical Association* 260 (1988): 2868.

5. Elizabeth McGlynn, et al., "The Quality of Health Care Delivered to Adults in the United States," *New England Journal of Medicine* 348 (June 26, 2003): 2635-2645. See also, Steven Asch, et al., "Who Is at Greatest Risk for Receiving Poor-Quality Health Care?" *New England Journal of Medicine* 354 (March 16, 2006): 1147–1156.

6. http://www.rand.org/pubs/working_papers/2006/RAND_WR174–1.pdf.

7. Statistics are taken from a Wikipedia article on heart attacks: http://en.wikipedia.org/wiki/Heart_attack .

8. Elizabeth McGlynn, et al., "Working Paper–Appendix, The Quality of Health Care Delivered to Adults in the United States," March 2006, accessible at http://www.rand.org/pubs/working_papers/2006/RAND_WR174–1.pdf, "CAD" section of paper, items 7 and 13.

9. McGlynn, "Working Paper," "CAD" section of paper, items 10 and 14.

10. McGlynn, "Working Paper," "CAD" section of paper, item 8.

11. McGlynn, "Working Paper," "CAD" section of paper, item 15.

12. All statistics in this paragraph come from Elizabeth McGlynn, et al., "The Quality of Health Care Delivered to Adults in the United States," *New England Journal of Medicine* 348 (June 26, 2003): 2635-2645, at page 2642.

13. See http://www.healthcentral.com/diabetes/type-II-diabetes-000060_10–145_5.html.

14. http://www.diabetes.org/whos-who-on-your-health-care-team/the-first-visit.jsp.

15. What RAND says every diabetic needs (taken from McGlynn, "Working Paper," Diabetes section):

1. Glycosylated hemoglobin (hemoglobin A1C) every 6 months.
2. Annual eye and visual exam.
3. Total serum cholesterol and HDL cholesterol tests documented.
4. Annual measurement of urine protein documented.
5. Foot examination at least twice a year.
6. Blood pressure measured at every visit.
7. Patients taking insulin should monitor their glucose at home unless documented to be unable or unwilling.
8. Newly diagnosed diabetics should receive dietary and exercise counseling.
9. Type 2 diabetics who have failed dietary therapy should receive oral hypoglycemic therapy.
10. Type 2 diabetics who have failed oral hypoglycemics should be offered insulin.
11. Diabetics with proteinuria should be offered an ACE inhibitor within 3 months of the notation of proteinuria unless contraindicated.
12. Patients with diabetes should have a follow-up visit at least every 6 months.

16. See the RAND list at http://www.rand.org/pubs/working_papers/2006/RAND_WR174–1.pdf.

Chapter 17

1. It's called the Josie King Foundation, http://www.josieking.org.

2. http://www.josieking.org/page.cfm?pageID=18.

3. Sue Sheridan, Nancy Conrad, Sorrel King, Jennifer Dingman, and Charles Denham, "Disclosure Through Our Eyes," *Journal of Patient Safety* 4.1 (2008): 18-26.

4. http://www.asahq.org/news/asanews042408.htm.

5. Sue Sheridan, Nancy Conrad, Sorrel King, Jennifer Dingman, and Charles Denham, "Disclosure Through Our Eyes," *Journal of Patient Safety* 4.1 (2008): 18-26.

6. Elizabeth McGlynn, et al., "The Quality of Health Care Delivered to Adults in the United States," *New England Journal of Medicine* 348 (June 26, 2003): 2635-2645.

7. Steven Asch, et al., "Who Is at Greatest Risk for Receiving Poor-Quality Health Care?" *New England Journal of Medicine* 354.11 (March 16, 2006): 1147-1156.

Epilogue

1. You can read more about the Lexington Veterans program at http://www.annals.org/cgi/reprint/131/12/963.pdf.

2. Here is a list of medical society ethics committees that help mediate fee disputes: http://www.ama-assn.org/ama/pub/category/13365.html.

3. You have to hunt diligently on the Web site to find how to make a formal complaint. Here's the page for D.C. and Maryland: http://www.delmarvafoundation.org/html/content_pages/Medicare_Connection/care_concerns.html, and the page for Virginia: http://www.vhqc.org/index/Exercise_Your_Rights.

4. Public Citizen, Inc. v. Department of Health and Human Services, 332 F.3d 654 (D.C. Cir. 2003).

5. These studies were gathered and analyzed by Philip G. Peters Jr. in his excellent article, "Doctors and Juries," *Michigan Law Review* 105.7 (May 2007): 1453-1495.

Index